Cosmo's Sexiest Beauty Secrets

The Ultimate Guide to Looking Gorgeous

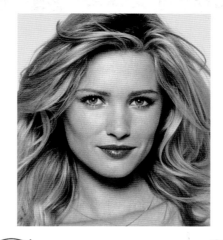

Cosmo's Sexiest Beauty Secrets

The Ultimate Guide to Looking Gorgeous

The Editors of COSMOPOLITAN

HEARST BOOKS

A division of Sterling Publishing Co., Inc.

New York / London

www.sterlingpublishing.com

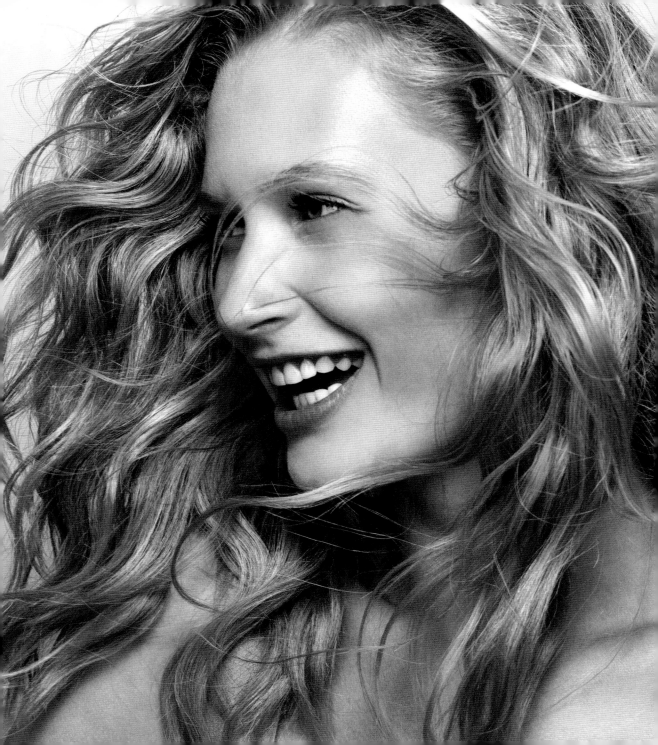

CONTENTS

6 INTRODUCTION What Is Sexy Beauty?
Cosmo's signature look is famously captivating.
It features sparkling eyes, shiny hair, and
soft skin—just for starters. Here, we define our
get-gorgeous formula.

8 SECRETS OF Gorgeous Skin
Looking beautiful starts with getting smooth,
clear, even-toned skin. Follow our maintenance
plan and your face will look absolutely amazing.

28 SECRETS OF A Flawless Face
A little bit of makeup manipulation can do
wonders to cover blemishes, even out
blotchiness, and hide under-eye circles. Whatever
the flaw is, our genius tricks resolve it.

44 SECRETS OF Mesmerizing Eyes
Your eyes aren't just the windows to your soul,
they are a weapon of seduction. Count on these
moves to get a hypnotic gaze.

66 SECRETS OF Alluring Lips
Few things are more enticing than a luscious
pair of lips. Our makeup techniques will
make your pout look full, pretty, and inviting.

84 SECRETS OF Amazing Hair
Find out how to make all that time you spend
on your hair worthwhile. There's brilliant
advice here on everything from daily care to
daring new styles and colors to try.

118 SECRETS OF A Sexy Body
Whether you're revealing just a hint of skin or
showing off your entire birthday suit, we
offer ways to get glowing from head to toe.

140 SECRETS OF Seductive Scent
Your scent can speak volumes about you and lure
a man by his nose. Ensure that your fragrance
is working up to its full potential with our tips.

156 SECRETS OF Perfect Nails
A glossy manicure is the quickest way to make
you look and feel glamorous. So buff up on
how to get your hands (and feet) in stellar shape.

170 SECRETS OF Spoiling Yourself
Spa-Style
Reap the blissful, beautifying benefits of a day
spent at a luxe spa right at home. We have
a slew of easy—yet indulgent—strategies.

182 BONUS SECRETS What Guys
Love (and Hate) About
Your Beauty Habits
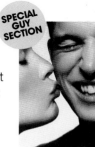
SPECIAL GUY SECTION

Not only do men *notice* your looks,
they have some strong opinions about
female primping practices. Read what
they have to say in their own words.

186 INDEX

190 PHOTO CREDITS

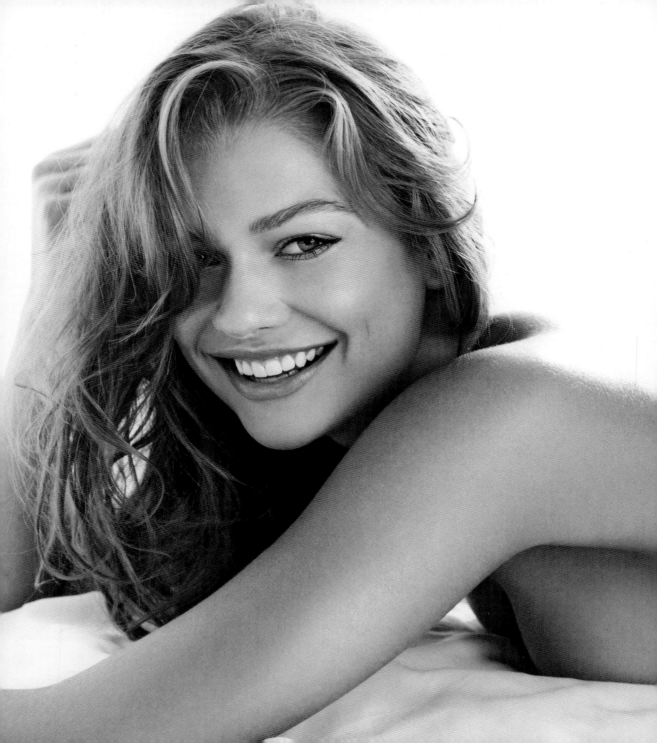

What Is Sexy Beauty?

Sexy beauty is an easy, inviting, and intoxicating look that plays up a woman's most sensuous traits.

Some defining qualities: healthy, shiny hair that has lots of body; silky, glowing skin that begs to be touched; full, smooth lips that can beckon a man from across the room; and smoky, smoldering eyes that captivate—in or out of the bedroom.

Looking and feeling sexy cultivates confidence, and in turn, that boost of self-esteem encourages you to make even more daring beauty moves, say by sporting fire engine red lips, taking a new hairstyle for a spin, or spritzing on an unapologetically sultry fragrance.

And who better than Cosmo to teach you the most seductive beauty tricks on the planet? Our book will give you everything you need to max out your innate sexiness. It's there just waiting to be unleashed.

Skin

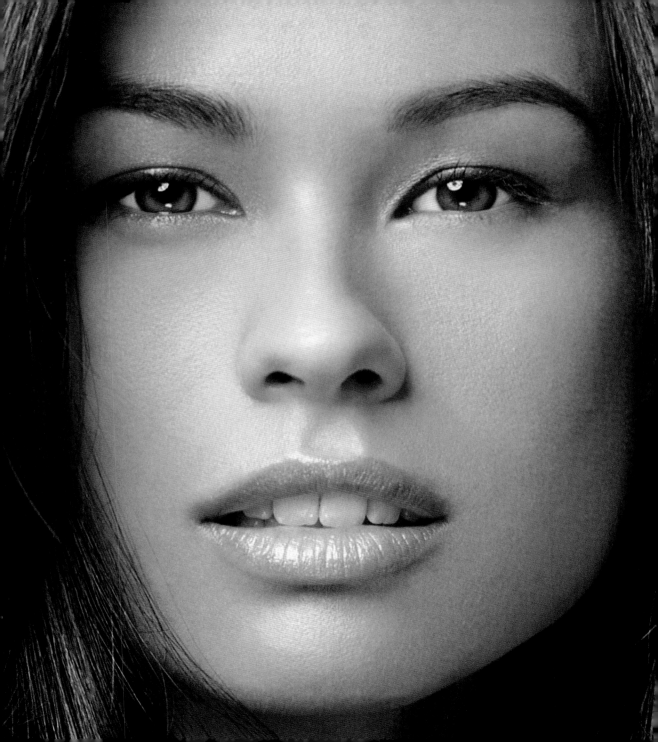

Gorgeous Skin

■ There are a few times when your face is pretty much guaranteed to look radiant: after a run, following a facial, and naturally, postsex. The rest of the time, you have to work at it a little, and that means adhering to a smart skin-care routine and, of course, being diligent about using sunscreen every day. "Your complexion glows when it's healthy, hydrated, and smooth," says New York City dermatologist Soren White. Read on to get the maintenance tips that will solve all your biggest skin woes and score you a beautiful complexion.

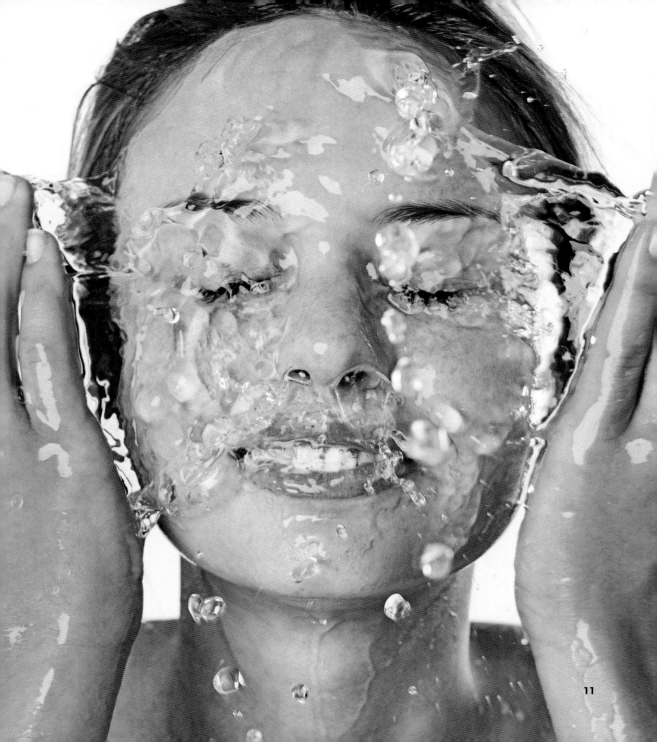

WHAT'S YOUR SKIN TYPE?

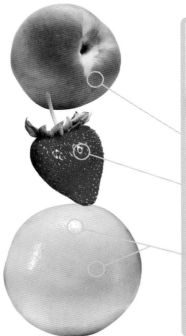

Even the most amazing products won't do squat if they're not meant for your skin type. We help you figure out what complexion category you fall into.

SKIN TYPE	CHARACTERISTICS
DRY	Small pores, dullness, skin feels tight postcleansing
OILY	Large pores, acne prone, frequently looks shiny
COMBINATION	Forehead, nose, and chin are oily while cheeks are drier
NORMAL	Similar to those of combination skin but with less oil in the T-zone area

SOURCE: NEW JERSEY COSMETIC DERMATOLOGIST CHRISTOPHER SCIALES

YOU SHOULD KNOW...
Three Ways to Max Out Moisturizer

1 Apply your cream to freshly washed damp skin within three minutes to seal in moisture that's already there. **2** Massage the cream in for at least 15 seconds to boost circulation and push the lotion as far into your skin as possible. **3** Screw the lid on tightly to prevent oxidation, which can decrease the potency of certain ingredients.

SOURCES: CALIFORNIA DERM AVA SHAMBAN; NEW YORK DERM DAVID BANK; MIAMI AND NYC DERM FREDRIC BRANDT

Daily Care for Every Type

Here's the basic cleansing and moisturizing regimen you should follow every day.

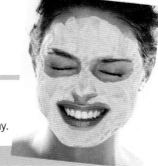

IF YOUR SKIN IS...	CLEANSING	MOISTURIZING
DRY	Wash with a mild, creamy, soap-free formula at night and just rinse with warm water in the morning.	Your skin can handle a cream that contains major hydrators like silicone, ceramides, or glycerin. They prevent moisture from escaping your skin.
OILY	Oily skin needs a potent cleanser with salicylic or alpha-hydroxy acid to get rid of dead skin and dissolve the excess sebum that plugs your pores.	Even if you don't feel you need it, you should use a moisturizer. Get a non-comedogenic (won't clog pores) one with a humectant (it attracts water from the air to your skin), such as sodium PCA, hyaluronic acid, or ceramides.
COMBINATION	An oil-free foaming cleanser with salicylic acid will get rid of the oil without stripping the dry areas.	If the dry parts are red and irritated, use a calming cream with chamomile or aloe. Otherwise, treat your skin as if it were oily with a humectant lotion.
NORMAL	Wash twice a day with a gentle soap-free, water-soluble formula.	Try out a bunch of lightweight noncomedogenic lotions until you find one that makes your skin feel its softest and smoothest.

SERVE YOURSELF RIGHT

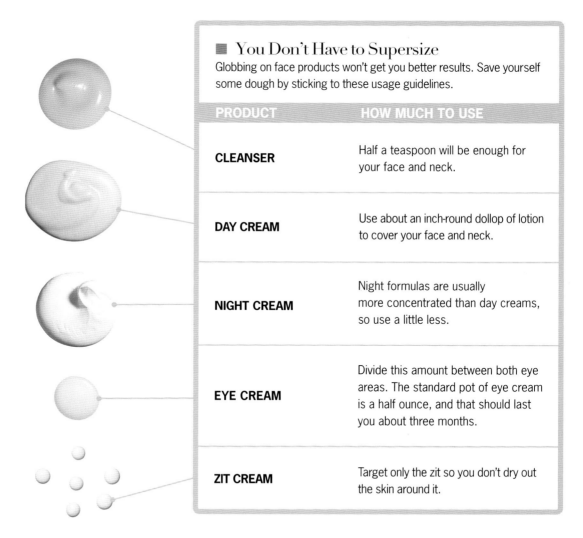

■ You Don't Have to Supersize

Globbing on face products won't get you better results. Save yourself some dough by sticking to these usage guidelines.

PRODUCT	HOW MUCH TO USE
CLEANSER	Half a teaspoon will be enough for your face and neck.
DAY CREAM	Use about an inch-round dollop of lotion to cover your face and neck.
NIGHT CREAM	Night formulas are usually more concentrated than day creams, so use a little less.
EYE CREAM	Divide this amount between both eye areas. The standard pot of eye cream is a half ounce, and that should last you about three months.
ZIT CREAM	Target only the zit so you don't dry out the skin around it.

Exfoliating Advice

Exfoliating is an absolute must since it boosts radiance, evens skin tone, unclogs pores, and diminishes fine lines. And since there are various ways you can slough, the trick is to pick a method that's right for your skin type, says cosmetic dermatologist Christopher Sciales. One rule that applies to everyone: Don't use a chemical peel or microdermabrasion product more than once a week, especially if your cleanser and face lotion already contain an exfoliating ingredient. "Overscrubbing can cause irritation and breakouts," says Dr. Sciales. Below, figure out which exfoliating method will work best for you.

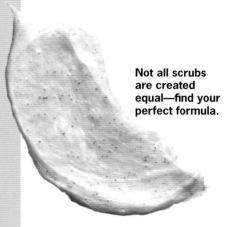

Not all scrubs are created equal—find your perfect formula.

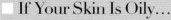 If Your Skin Is Oily...

You can use an exfoliating face wash on acne-prone skin every day as long as the formula is meant for daily use. You can also try an at-home microdermabrasion kit—a more intense method of physical scrubbing that uses aluminum or salt crystals—once a week to help diminish the appearance of acne scars and large pores.

If Your Skin Is Normal or Dry...

Normal and dry complexions can be buffed two or three times per week with a mild microbead scrub (the synthetic balls are more gentle than ones that contain ground-up nuts or seeds). You should avoid microdermabrasion, which can be too harsh for your skin, and instead use a store-bought alpha-hydroxy chemical peel (such as one that contains glycolic and lactic acids) once a week.

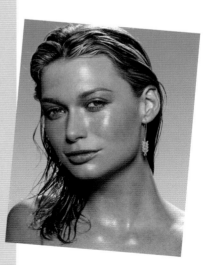

YOUR PRACTICE-SAFE-SUN PLAN

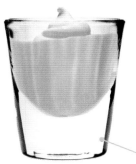

A shot glass's worth of SPF lotion is all you need to cover your whole bod.

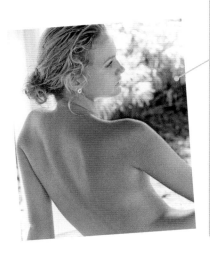

The most important thing you can do to maintain the beauty of your skin is to protect it from UV light. The sun's rays can trigger dark spots, wrinkles, and even skin cancer. We know you're following some basic rules (covering up at the beach and skipping tanning beds), but you may need to step up your SPF routine. Start with this advice.

- **Put the lotion on 15 to 30 minutes before going outdoors.** This gives the sunscreen enough time to be absorbed into your skin and offer you ultimate protection.

- **Squeeze out an ounce and a half—the amount to fill an average shot glass.** "Coat your body in a thin, even layer; there's no need to frost yourself like a cupcake," explains Noah S. Heftler, MD, clinical instructor in dermatology at Weill Medical College.

- **Apply it all over.** Put the sunscreen on while you're completely naked so you can apply it everywhere. Then, when your swimsuit moves around, the skin that gets exposed is still protected. Make sure your legs and upper back are covered; melanoma most often strikes these body areas in women.

- **Be gentle to your face.** It's fine to use the same product you use for your body, but if your face is prone to breakouts, invest in a sunscreen specially formulated to prevent blemishes.

- **Reapply every two hours** if you are lazing around outside and every 30 minutes if you're doing something active that's causing you to sweat, even if the label says it's waterproof.

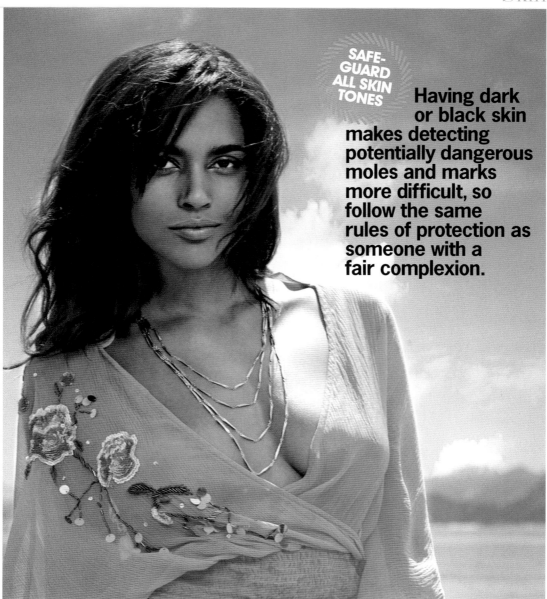

SAFE-GUARD ALL SKIN TONES Having dark or black skin makes detecting potentially dangerous moles and marks more difficult, so follow the same rules of protection as someone with a fair complexion.

FIGHT AGING—STARTING NOW

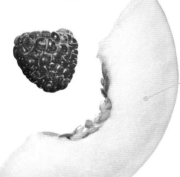

These fruits have a hefty dose of skin-pleasing antioxidants.

Studies show that the way you take care of your face in your 20s and early 30s is a key factor in how it ages over time. Here, what you can do to keep your skin looking perpetually youthful.

Try a retinoid. Vitamin-A derivatives (known as retinoids) exfoliate as well as stimulate collagen production so your skin looks plumper, smoother, and firmer. You can try an OTC version or ask your derm for Renova, a stronger prescription formula. Retinoids break down in sunlight and can be very drying, so use it at night twice a week with a mild moisturizer over it. Slowly work up to applying it every night. If your skin is too sensitive for these powerful potions, try a weekly at-home glycolic-acid peel.

Add antioxidants. When applied topically in the form of a serum or lotion, antioxidants neutralize free radicals caused by UV rays and other skin-damaging environmental factors. Research shows that you'll get even more protection if you use a product containing a cocktail of antioxidants, so look for one that contains a blend of vitamins C and E, plus ferulic acid or green tea.

Nourish at night. Skin does a better job of absorbing moisturizers overnight than during the day. Choose ones with collagen stimulators like pentapeptides, retinol, or alpha-hydroxy acids.

Treat your eyes. If you're not using eye cream already, get going. The skin around your eyes is the thinnest and least oily so it shows signs of aging first.

SOURCES: MIAMI DERMATOLOGIST LESLIE BAUMANN, NEW JERSEY DERMATOLOGIST JEANINE DOWNIE, AND NYC DERMATOLOGIST CHERYL KARCHER

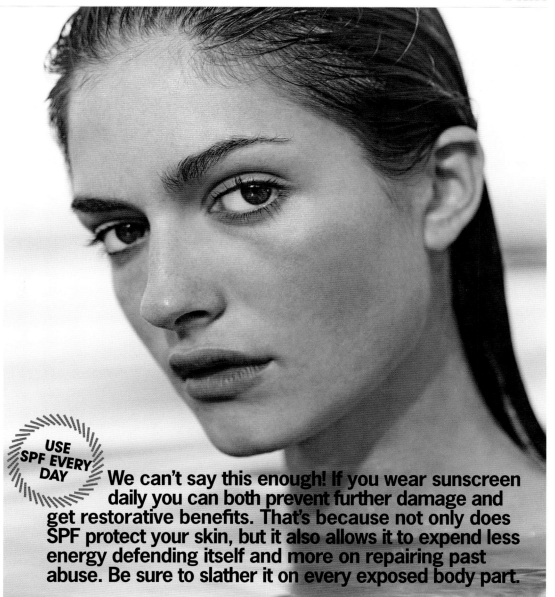

USE SPF EVERY DAY We can't say this enough! If you wear sunscreen daily you can both prevent further damage and get restorative benefits. That's because not only does SPF protect your skin, but it also allows it to expend less energy defending itself and more on repairing past abuse. Be sure to slather it on every exposed body part.

YOUR SKIN'S BIGGEST AGING ISSUE

Here, the skin concern that plagues each of the

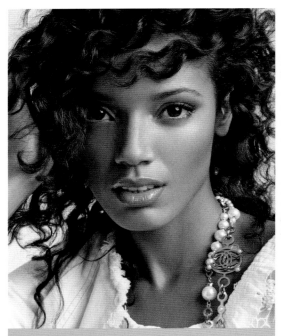

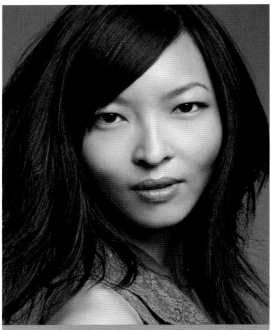

◼ African-Americans

KEY CONCERN: Hyperpigmentation
Black skin's high melanin levels can cause dark under-eye circles and acne scars.

SOLUTION: Get an eye cream with vitamin A, C, E, or K. Chemical peels or microdermabrasion will fade dark marks on the rest of your face.

◼ Asians

KEY CONCERN: Sunspots
Porcelain, milky skin is prone to freckles and brown spots from sun exposure.

SOLUTION: Stay in the shade, wear SPF 30 every day, and try a botanical-based or prescription fade cream to make sunspots less noticeable.

following ethnicities the most

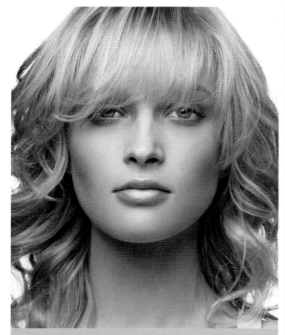 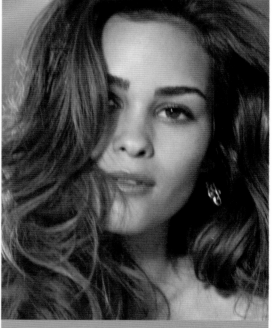

■ Caucasians

KEY CONCERN: Wrinkles and redness
The lighter the skin, the more susceptible it is to irritation and sun damage.

SOLUTION: Use a night cream with alpha-hydroxy acids or retinol to speed up cell turnover. Calm ruddy skin with a soothing chamomile face cream.

■ Hispanics

KEY CONCERN: Unevenness
Medium skin can turn blotchy from sun damage quickly.

SOLUTION: Be diligent about protecting your natural honey-toned glow. Using SPF 30 every day should do the trick.

EAT, DRINK, AND SNOOZE YOUR WAY TO GLOWIER SKIN

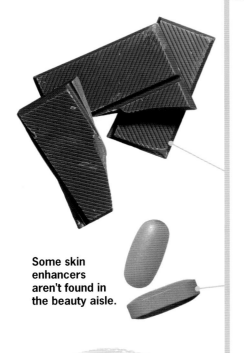

Some skin enhancers aren't found in the beauty aisle.

All those potions and lotions in your bathroom cabinet are great at warding off lines and wrinkles, but there are some less obvious ways to score an ageless complexion.

- **Eat more omega-3-rich foods.** Studies show that the omega-3 fatty acids found in fresh catches, such as salmon, mackerel, and albacore tuna, maintain skin's moisture, keeping it luminous. Not a seafood lover? Try walnuts, flaxseed, tofu, or pop a fish-oil supplement, says Alan C. Logan, coauthor of *The Clear Skin Diet*.

- **Have some chocolate too.** The flavanol antioxidant in cocoa can create smoother, less scaly skin, according to researchers—sweet news, right? Mix pure cocoa powder into your morning smoothie or top your salad with flavanol-rich fruits (apples and blueberries are prime picks).

- **Take your vitamins.** It won't work overnight, but a regular multivitamin delivers a whole slew of nutrients (specifically zinc, iron, and vitamin A) that keep your skin, hair, and nails healthy and glowing in the long term, says cosmetic derm Christopher Sciales.

- **Sleep is essential.** Regular exercise increases blood flow to the surface of your skin, and just think of all the fun ways you can work up a sweat. At some point, though, you'll need shut-eye. So if you're getting less than seven hours every night, your skin will pay the price, says Dr. Sciales.

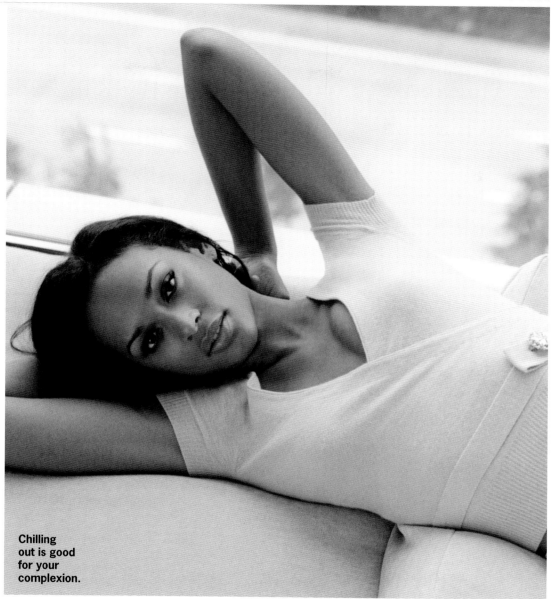

Chilling
out is good
for your
complexion.

Never Get a Pimple Again

You thought acne would beat it for good when you hit your 20s. So why in the world are you still breaking out? Well, derms say that modern chicks have a slew of new acne-causing factors in their lives like stress, elevated male hormones (especially women who work in competitive environments), and misinformation about treating adult acne. Keep reading and we'll tell you what to do depending on the severity of your situation.

CLEAR THE PATH TO GREAT SKIN

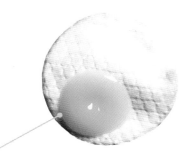

▰ Dealing With Mild to Moderate Acne

This three-pronged attack should end annoying breakouts.

Cleansers. Look for a mild face wash that's oil-free and noncomedogenic. Avoid anything that's overly drying, since that could cause your skin to rebound by producing excess oil.

Moisturizers. Choose an oil-free lotion that contains salicylic acid (which loosens stuffed pores) and retinol (which trains your skin to shed dead cells properly).

Spot treatments. Buy one with a 2 percent concentration of salicylic acid or a 10 percent concentration of benzoyl peroxide. Those are the strongest amounts you can get without a Rx. Dab it on your pimple with a cotton swab so you don't spread bacteria.

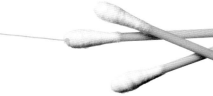

Breakouts begone! A simple daily strategy can keep skin free of spots.

YOU SHOULD KNOW...

Freeze Out a Zit

If despite your best efforts you still get a pimple, hide it like this: Dab toner over the zit to dry up excess oil, then cool and flatten the bump with an ice cube (wrapped in a tissue) for one minute. "Don't leave the cube on too long or you'll wind up with redness," Los Angeles clinical aesthetician Sonya Dakar warns. Last, use a spot-treatment product before dotting on concealer.

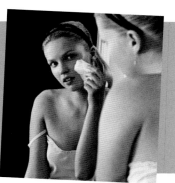

HELP FOR SEVERE ACNE

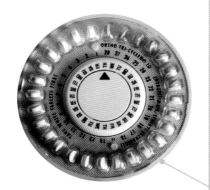

If you can't get your skin under control on your own, talk to your derm about these treatments.

Retinoid creams. A prescription-strength retinol product, like Ziana, Differin, Tazorac, or Retin-A, can help purge the dirt and oil that's clogging up your pores.

Oral antibiotics. Meds like Solodyn, Doxycycline, Minocycline, and Tetracycline kill the acne-causing bacteria in the hair follicle and reduce swelling.

Birth-control pills. If excessive hormones are the culprit, the right birth-control pill (typically one with a combo of estrogen and progestin) can normalize their levels and prevent breakouts.

Accutane. For cystic acne, consider Accutane, a vitamin-A derivative that stops the oil glands from producing acne-causing sebum. A word of warning, however: The drug has serious side effects and cannot be taken if you're pregnant or could become pregnant.

In-office treatments. The newest laser—Isolaz—kills bacteria painlessly and extracts gunk from pores. However, it costs $500 per session, and you'll need four or five 10-minute sessions spaced a month apart with touch-ups every six months to maintain results. Other derm-administered procedures: Chemical peels, which clean out pores and reduce inflammation, and blue-light therapy, which helps kill bacteria and shrink the size of the sebaceous glands.

SOURCE: DERMATOLOGIST FREDRIC BRANDT

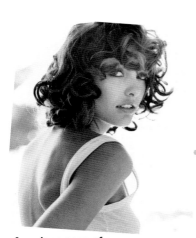

A serious case of acne may call for a high-tech solution.

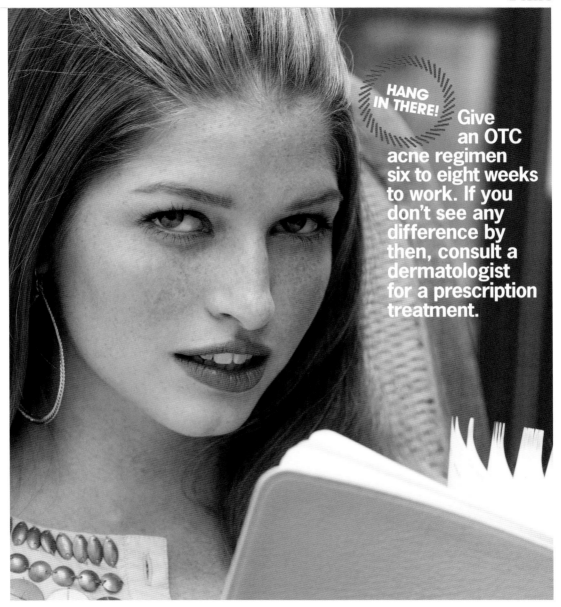

HANG IN THERE! Give an OTC acne regimen six to eight weeks to work. If you don't see any difference by then, consult a dermatologist for a prescription treatment.

Face

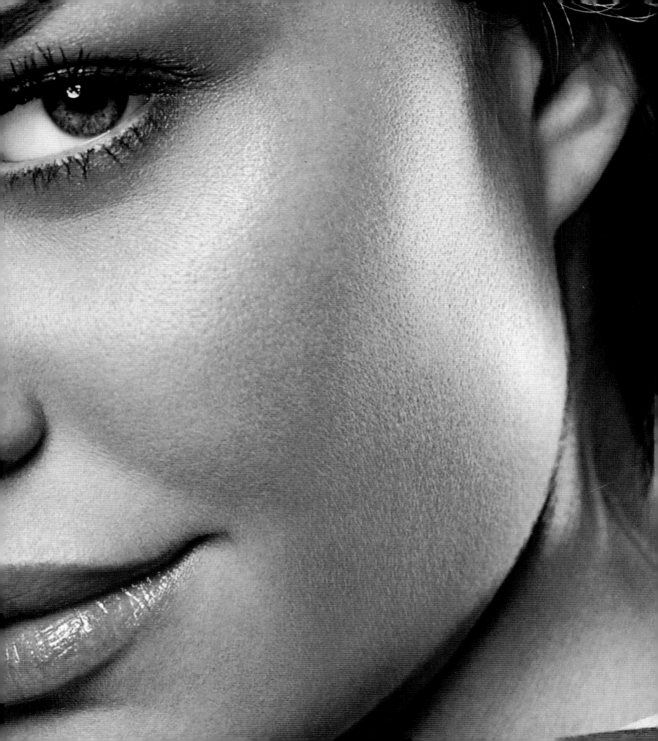

A Flawless Face

■ Every chick on the planet (yes, even models) has face flaws. Thankfully, a little bit of makeup manipulation can do wonders to hide blemishes, even out your skin tone, and brighten dark under-eye circles. As you'll hear over and over, a key part of faking an amazing complexion is finding the right makeup shade for your skin tone, whether it be foundation, bronzer, or blush. Here, all you need to know to look absolutely luminous.

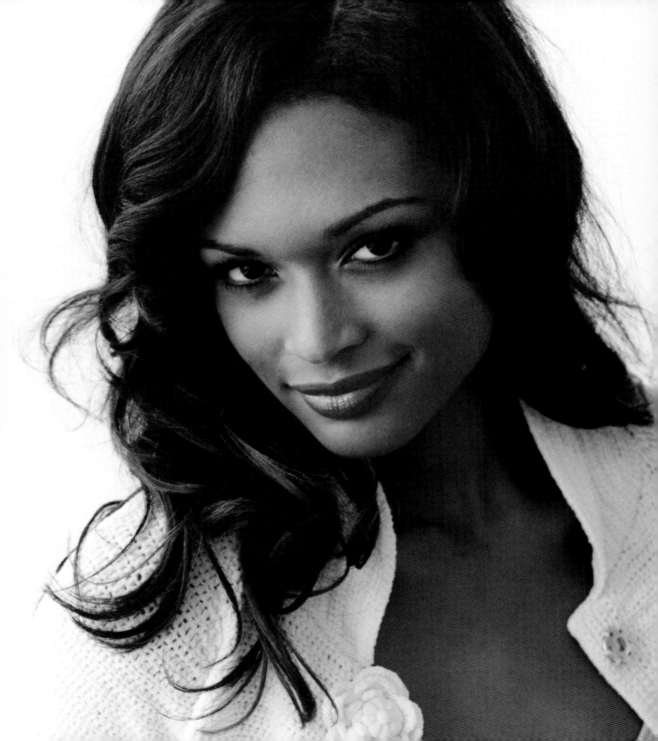

FIND THE RIGHT FOUNDATION SHADE

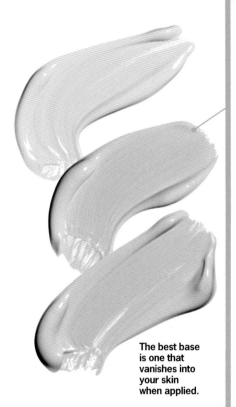

The best base is one that vanishes into your skin when applied.

Applying an undetectable base is the first step in achieving a gorgeous face. Here's help for picking your perfect hue.

■ **If you're shopping at a department store…**
Swipe three possible matches on your lower cheek or jawline (the shade should closely match your neck as well as your face). Take a mirror and head toward a window or go outside so you can see the hues in natural light. The one that fades into your skin without much blending is the winner, says celebrity makeup artist Carol Shaw, creator of LORAC Cosmetics.

■ **If you're shopping at the drugstore…**
The trick is to first determine if you are pale, medium, or dark. Once you know your skin tone, use the bottle shade name as a guideline. Pale skin tends to have some redness, so it's best to stay away from pink-toned foundation shades. Look for a hue labeled beige or buff to neutralize ruddiness. Girls in the middle of the skin-tone spectrum have light beige, olive, or tan complexions with warm undertones. Asian skin also falls into this category since it has a lot of yellow in it. Stick with shades labeled warm, medium, or golden. Dark skin can range from as light as cafe au lait to as deep as ebony. To prevent a grayish cast, go for colors like tan, sable, or chestnut. Also, African-American women often have oily skin, which can cause their base to oxidize and appear darker when it mixes with oil, so try a foundation that is slightly lighter than your complexion.

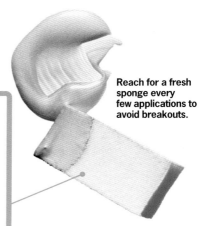

Reach for a fresh sponge every few applications to avoid breakouts.

■ Key Application Tips

● Clean fingers can provide the sheerest, most natural effect since the warmth of your hands helps to "melt" the base onto your skin, says NYC makeup artist Troy Surratt. It's best to use your fingers with liquid and cream foundation formulas.

● Sponges provide more coverage and are good for blending cream-to-powder or thicker liquid foundations. Tap, don't rub, the base into your face with the sponge for an even finish, says London makeup artist Jemma Kidd, founder of Jemma Kidd Make Up.

● A foundation brush gives a heavier, more velvety finish because you're literally painting on a liquid or cream base, says celebrity makeup pro Bobbi Brown, CEO of Bobbi Brown Cosmetics. This is ideal if you're going for a very polished look.

94%
of women would not cancel a date over a zit.
SOURCE: COSMO WEB POLL

YOU SHOULD KNOW...

Camouflage 101

A single concealer won't cut it on every area of your face. You need one with yellow or even green undertones for tackling the redness in a zit, plus a pink-tinged shade to counteract the blue in under-eye circles, says Kidd.

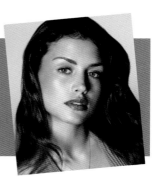

YOUR FOUNDATION WARDROBE

You should possess a few base formulas—from sheer to medium coverage—so you can choose depending on what's up with your skin. Here's what we recommend.

FOR DAYS WHEN...	GO FOR...
You need minimal help.	A liquid foundation or tinted moisturizer. They are sheer, blend easily, and will even out your skin tone. Look for versions that have light-reflecting pigments if you want to boost glow.
You have some obvious red splotches.	A cream-to-powder formula. It'll give you medium coverage and a noncakey finish.
You won't be able to touch up your makeup all day.	A transferproof base—it forms a light, flexible film that ensures the pigment won't fade for hours. Quick tip: Let your moisturizer absorb before applying your base, then blot your face with a tissue to remove any excess.
Your face is breaking out or you're more oily.	An oil-free foundation that contains the zit-fighting ingredient salicylic acid (it will say so on the package) won't clog pores or slide off your face.

YOU SHOULD KNOW...

Which goes on first: foundation or concealer?

FOUNDATION. "It's the base for everything," says New York City celebrity makeup artist Tina Turnbow. **"It evens out skin tone, so you can really see where, or if, you need concealer."**

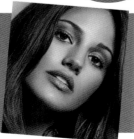

Get More From Your Base

- Mix your foundation with an equal part face lotion to create a tinted moisturizer.

- Blend foundation over your eyelids to hide tiny red blood vessels. It'll also serve as a base for your shadow.

- Use the foundation that pools and thickens in the bottle cap as a concealer in a pinch.

SWEETEN
YOUR CHEEKS

The key to faking killer cheekbones: Contour with two shades of blush.

■ A Lasting Flush

When you apply blush on bare skin it's likely to fade away fast. The trick is to prep your skin with a sheer layer of foundation and a light dusting of powder first, says makeup artist Carol Shaw. Both provide a base for the color to adhere to. Also, keep in mind that powder formulas have more staying power than cream versions while liquid and gel stains are pretty much budge-proof.

■ Master the Blush Stroke

A big, fluffy powder brush works well when you want to swoosh color all over, but when it comes to contouring, use a small, flat one instead since it allows more control, says makeup artist Jemma Kidd. To sculpt your cheeks, sweep a shimmery pink blush over the apples, then apply a matte bronze shade in the hollows. "This makes your cheekbones appear more prominent," says Kidd.

SEXY SECRET
Under-the-Radar Blush Zones

Sure, a rosy tint on cheeks enlivens a complexion...but why stop there? Dust a shimmery, pink powder over your upper cheekbones, eyelids, and hairline for an allover flush, says Cristina Bartolucci, cofounder and creative director of DuWop Cosmetics.

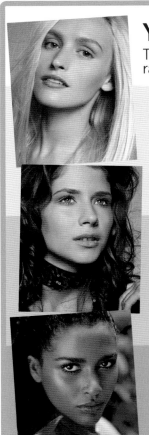

Your Prettiest Hue

The right shade of blush makes you look healthy and radiant. Here's what to look for based on your skin tone.

■ Fair Skin

If you have yellow undertones, go for a peachy blush. Complexions with cool, bluish undertones look best in soft pinks.

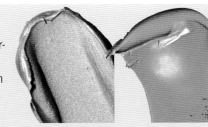

■ Medium Skin

Use a deep golden pink shade for a subtle day look. Pump it up at night with a vibrant apricot blush.

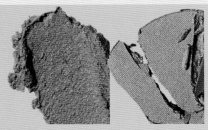

■ Dark Skin

You need colors that will pop against your skin. Rich plum or bright fuchsia will do the trick.

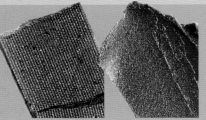

LOOK GREAT IN ANY LIGHT

Even the most beautiful makeup can look bad in the wrong lighting. Follow these tips and you'll be sitting pretty in every exposure.

■ When You're Indoors

Fluorescent light (found in indoor spaces) has a greenish cast, which can turn skin sallow, says L'Oréal consulting makeup artist Collier Strong. Cancel out this effect with a bright rose blush.

■ When You're in a Candlelit Room

The glow of a candle evens out skin tone and softens features, says Strong. Play up that luminosity by mixing a dollop of pearly lotion with a sheer foundation. (Skip bronzers, which can look muddy.) The shimmer will pick up the flecks of light thrown off by the flame.

■ When You're Outdoors

Everything is magnified in natural light, including blush, which can look overdone outside. Smashbox makeup artist Holly Mordini recommends using a cream or gel formula, which blends into skin more seamlessly and naturally than dark powders do.

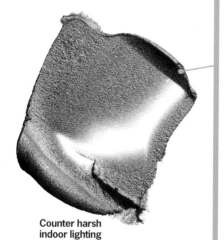

Counter harsh indoor lighting with a rosy blush hue.

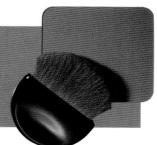

SEXY SECRET

Try a Bold Color

A bright flush mimics the rush of blood to the cheeks that occurs during orgasm, explains anthropologist Lionel Tiger, PhD. "Men see it as a sign of sexual readiness and react subconsciously."

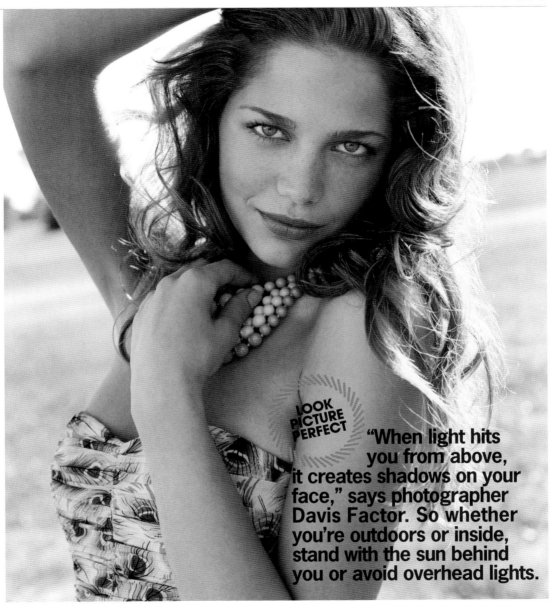

LOOK PICTURE PERFECT

"When light hits you from above, it creates shadows on your face," says photographer Davis Factor. So whether you're outdoors or inside, stand with the sun behind you or avoid overhead lights.

THE BEST BRONZER

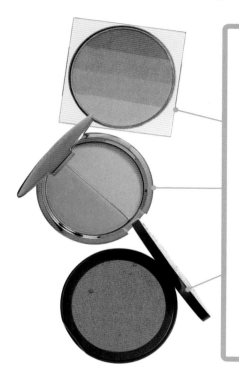

Bronzer can give you a sexy sun-kissed look (without any sun-induced damage). Plus, it's more user-friendly than self-tanner. For the most believable glow, use a shade that works with your skin tone, says New York City makeup artist Matin. Here's how to select the right one.

● **If you're fair with yellow undertones,** look for a palette that has a combination of warm peach, apricot, and bronze shades—it'll warm up your complexion without overpowering it.

● **If you're fair with pink undertones,** use both bronzer and blush to get the most natural effect. Dust a medium bronze shade over your forehead, nose, and cheeks first, then sweep a bright pink blush just on the apples of your cheeks.

● **If you have olive to dark skin,** you can pull off deeper hues like terra-cotta and copper. Apply it only where the sun naturally hits (cheekbones, nose, forehead), since an allover monotone hue looks fake. Hot tip: When dusted on cheekbones, a shimmery bronzer acts as a highlighter on African-American skin.

Get Your Gleam On

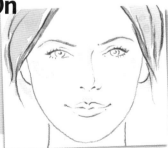

Your cheeks aren't fully dressed for a night out without highlighter. This shimmery liquid or powder makes you look bathed in candlelight...even when you're nowhere near a flame. It comes in a range of shades, but a pale gold hue gives an ethereal glow to all skin tones, says London makeup artist Charlotte Tilbury. Blend it on light-attracting areas including cheekbones, the bridge of your nose, brow bones, and right above your lips.

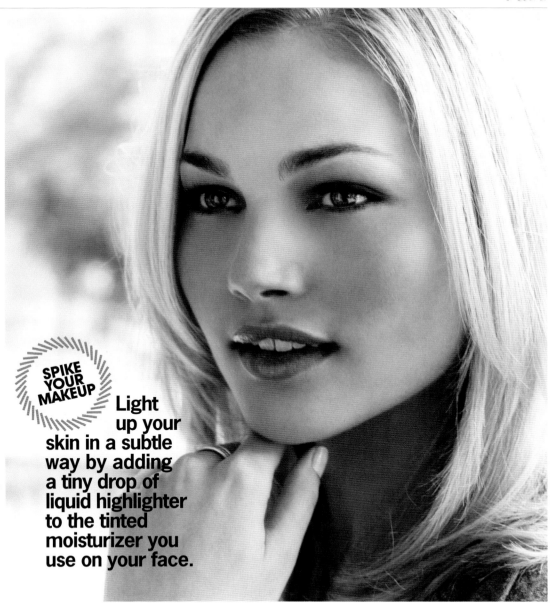

SPIKE YOUR MAKEUP Light up your skin in a subtle way by adding a tiny drop of liquid highlighter to the tinted moisturizer you use on your face.

BE A STUNNER ALL DAY LONG

The same makeup MO doesn't always work for both day and night. Here are expert tricks

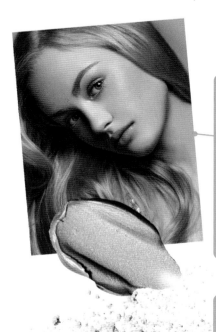

Weekday A.M.

Pretty and Polished

Smooth skin. When you wake up, your skin is in its most dewy state, so you don't need to cover it up much, says NYC dermatologist Francesca Fusco. Just apply a thin veil of a sheer foundation. Then dab a creamy concealer over blemishes and under-eye circles.

Rosy cheeks. Because your circulation is slower in the morning, your cheeks will look kind of pale, says Dr. Fusco. Amp up your flush factor with **cream blush**, then swirl on a powder bronzer for a subtle boost.

Weekday P.M.

Gorgeous and Glowy

Silky skin. By night your skin is dehydrated, says Dr. Fusco. Reach for a moisturizing foundation to look fresh. Then hide blemishes with concealer and dust shiny spots with a light layer of powder.

Gleaming cheeks. Ever notice how your face seems to get ruddy as the day goes on? Stress and caffeine intake can create extra redness by causing blood vessels to swell and expand under the skin, says Dr. Fusco. So don't pile on more blush—just brighten your existing shade with a sweep of **gold shimmer powder**.

that'll keep your face looking gorgeous around the clock.

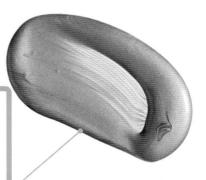

Weekend A.M.

Bronzed and Breezy

Sun-kissed skin. Extra sleep on the weekend helps boost blood flow, making under-eye circles less obvious. So just use a tinted moisturizer with SPF and top it off with liquid **bronzer.**

Radiant cheeks. Chances are, you're already rosy, since you're getting more heart-pumping activity (like power shopping) than during the week, notes Dr. Fusco. Play up your natural flush with a hint of cream blush on the apples of your cheeks.

Weekend P.M.

Seductive and Sexy

Iridescent skin. After the sun goes down, it's prime time to connect with guys. That means you'll want to reveal more of yourself, skin included. To really glow, apply shimmer powder on key areas—the brow bone, cheekbones, and décolletage.

Tawny cheeks. Adjust to the darkness of your surroundings with a **more dramatic blush** than you'd wear during the day. But apply it *before* you go out. Bar lighting tends to be cavelike, so you could overdo it by accident.

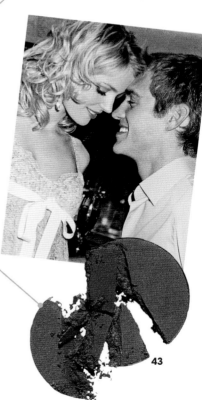

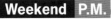

43

Eyes

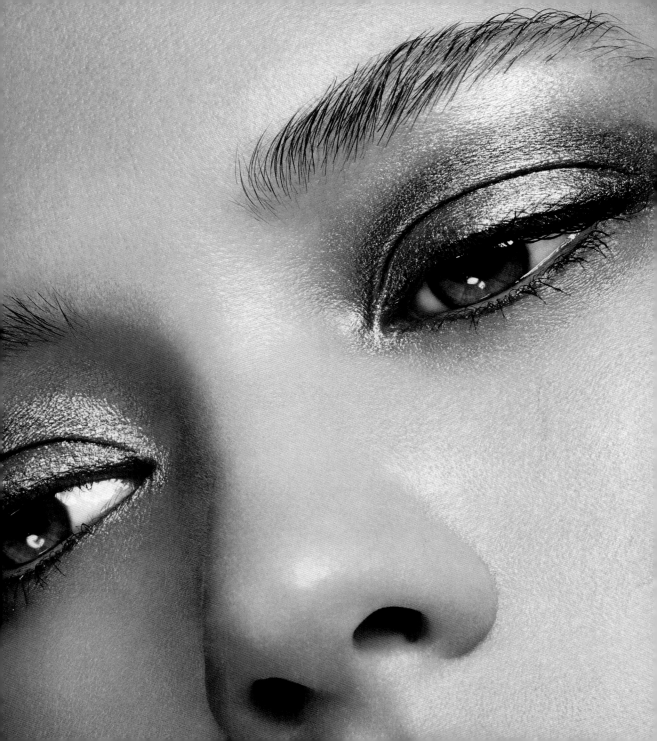

Mesmerizing Eyes

■ Your eyes are your most magnetic feature—and that's not *just* a reference to their beauty. They actually possess the ability to draw someone to you. "Attraction between two people begins with a gaze," says anthropologist David B. Givens, PhD. "When you feel a connection, your pupils dilate, which is a signal to guys to come closer." What's more, enhancing your orbs with makeup conveys confidence because it says that you want people to look at you. Here, you'll learn how to make your peepers look their biggest, brightest, and most captivating. Behold the tantalizing tricks....

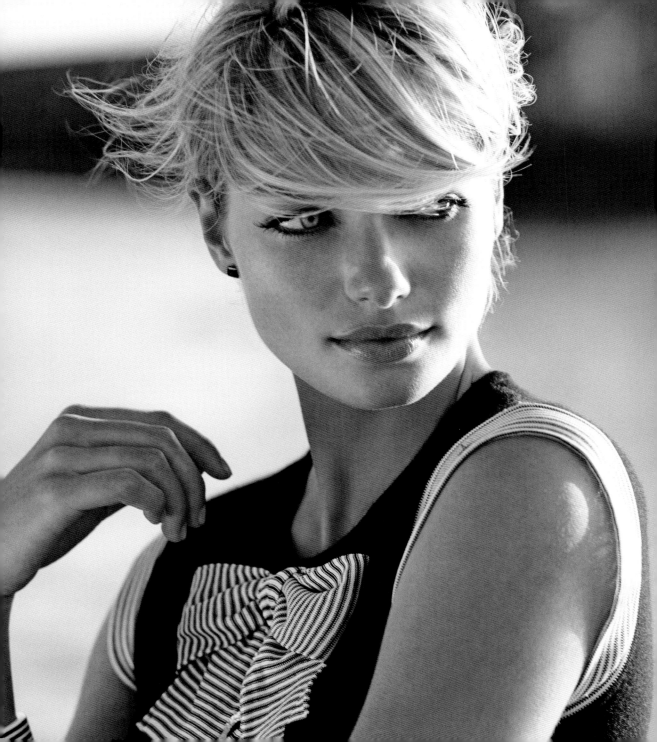

HOW TO FIND YOUR BEST COLORS

It's fun to experiment with trendy shadows, but you should have go-to hues that always give you gorgeous results. To figure out what they are, pick a shade that's opposite your eye color on the color wheel. "Using contrasting colors is a great way to enhance your eyes," says makeup pro Cristina Bartolucci. Here's how to use this trick to make your irises sparkle.

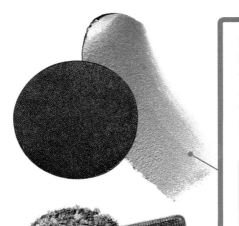

GREEN EYES

Green-eyed girls can make their eyes look piercing with a plum or warm lavender shade, since both are on the periphery of the red color family, which is almost green's opposite. However, you should avoid true red shadows (like brick or burgundy) or you'll overwhelm your eyes rather than play up their hue.

BLUE EYES

To highlight the natural beauty of blue eyes, use a shadow that has hints of the opposite color family: orange. This group includes earthy colors like chocolate, bronze, and gold as well as neutral colors like taupe and punchier shades like tangerine.

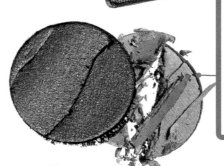

BROWN EYES

Brown eyes look hot in a slew of shades. But to make chocolate peepers really pop, swipe on a blue-based shadow. Since blue is in the closest opposite color family, it makes brown eyes look stunning. Choose a rich cobalt, navy, or violet.

Make a Stellar Shadow Purchase

There's more to buying an eye shadow than picking out a fabulous color—the product should be well-made so it'll create the most flawless, long-lasting look. When shopping for a new shadow, smear it on the back of your hand, advises Maureen Kelly, creator of Tarte Cosmetics. If it's high quality, the shadow will glide easily across your skin without skipping and create an even coat of color. Also, it should feel silky smooth, not grainy. A rough texture is a sign it will clump on your lids, especially if your creases tend to be oily.

3 WAYS TO MAKE YOUR EYE EFFECT LAST LONGER

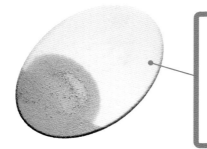

■ Prep Your Orbs

If you just slap eye makeup on naked lids, it'll fade within a few hours. Instead, first blend a shadow primer over your whole eye area—lids and inner and outer corners. It gives your shadow something to grab onto, plus the color will show up even better, says Wende Zomnir, creative director of Urban Decay Cosmetics.

The Eye-shadow Quad—Demystified

Figuring out where to apply each of the four colors in a shadow palette is on par with solving a Sudoku puzzle. Not anymore. Here's where to put what.

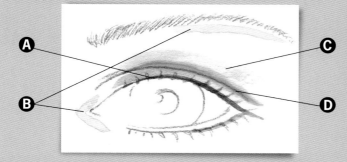

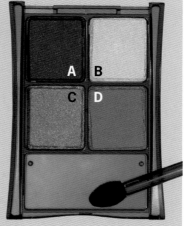

A Use the deepest hue to define your lash lines.

B Highlight brow bones and the inner corners of your eyes with the lightest shimmery shade.

C Sweep the second palest color all over your lids.

D Blend the medium tone into your creases (but not above them) to add definition and depth.

■ Go for a Stay-Put Texture

Need an eye makeup that can withstand a heat wave (or a marathon mattress session)? Choose an eye shadow that goes on creamy but dries to a powder finish. "These formulas won't rub off," says makeup artist Holly Mordini. As for liner, stroke on one that contains nylon-12, an ingredient that gives the pencil staying power.

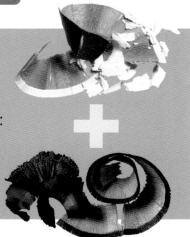

Eye-shadow creams that turn to powders are budge-proof.

■ Last-All-Night Lashes

For fringe that looks as seductive at sunrise as it did when you first hit the party, apply a couple coats of waterproof mascara—even if you won't be anywhere near a pool, Jacuzzi, or rainstorm.

SEXY SECRET

Eye-Enlarging Trick

No matter what shape your peepers are, this beauty move will make them appear alluringly larger: Rim the insides of your eyelids with white liner, says celeb makeup artist Polly Osmond. Then define the upper and lower lashes with a charcoal liner. Finish with three coats of black mascara.

SULTRY EVENING EYES

Look sexy—no matter where the night takes you.

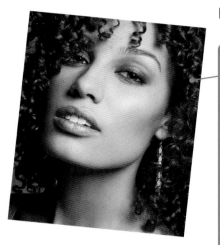

■ Hitting a Club

To get an intense come-hither look, pat on three coats of cream shadow in a metallic hue (like copper or pewter). Before putting the color on, dust your lids with translucent powder to prevent the shadow from building up in your creases.

■ Going on a Romantic Date

You know how the light from a flickering flame makes your eyes look all glowy? Intensify that effect by dotting a shimmery pink shadow in the center of your lids. Since this is the roundest part of your eyelid, the glimmer will reflect the light, creating an illuminated look.

You Can Pull Off a Vibrant Hue

Intense shadow shades can be scary (*Teal? Really?*). But you're not the type to shy away from being bold. Below, L.A. makeup artist Robin Siegel tackles the challenge.

1 Use a thin liner brush to rim only the outer corner of your eye, right at the roots of your lashes. Then blend the shadow along the entire length of your lower lash line.

2 Sweep a light coat of shadow onto your lid and up into the crease to create a subtle hint of color. Next, wet your liner brush and dip it into the shadow (the water will make the color look darker). Position the brush on the outer corner of your upper lash line and wiggle it along your lashes toward your inner corner. This will give the eye definition and depth.

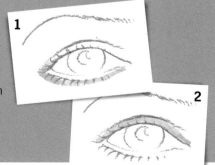

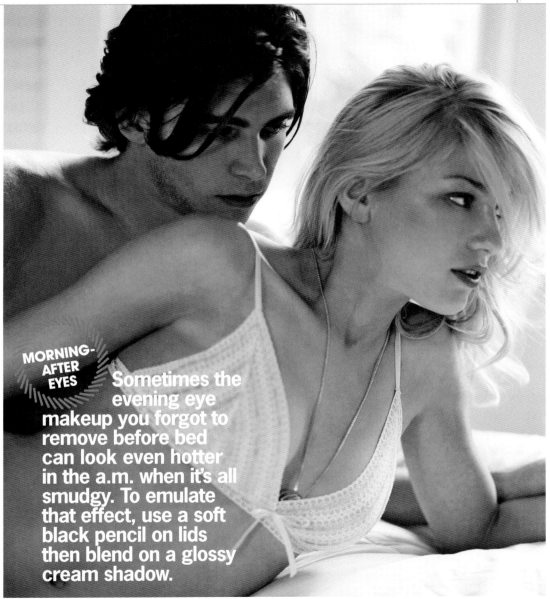

MORNING-AFTER EYES Sometimes the evening eye makeup you forgot to remove before bed can look even hotter in the a.m. when it's all smudgy. To emulate that effect, use a soft black pencil on lids then blend on a glossy cream shadow.

TONS OF EYE-ENHANCING MOVES

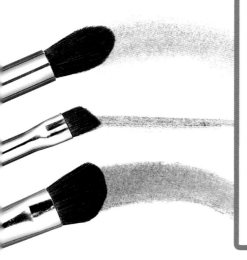

■ One Hue, Three Sexy Effects

Did you know that your favorite eye shadow is capable of creating more than one look? Here's how to make a hue multitask.

1 Give your lids a sheer wash of color by lightly dabbing a dry fluffy brush into the shadow and blending it from lashes to creases.

2 Get dramatic, defined eyes by running a small, stiff liner brush through the shadow then rimming your lashes.

3 If you're going for a bold, notice-me effect, dampen your brush slightly before dipping it into the shadow. The water will intensify the color for a deeper payoff.

YOU SHOULD KNOW...

Pick the Perfect Tool

Using the right shadow brush makes a huge difference when whipping up any eye look. Here's the deal: Shorter-bristled versions give more control and accuracy, so they're best for lining and defining, says celebrity makeup artist Mally Roncal. Longer-bristled ones are softer and less precise, making them better for blending and subtle effects.

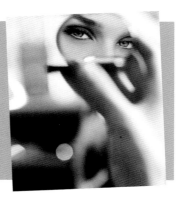

Tips for Every Eye Shape

SMALL EYES

Supersize eyes with light shadows (dark colors can be minimizing). If you use liner, just do the top lid. Another trick: "Sweep mascara on your upper lashes and only the center of your lower lashes," says New York City makeup artist Ramy Gafni. This will draw attention to the center of your eye, which is the roundest—and therefore widest—part.

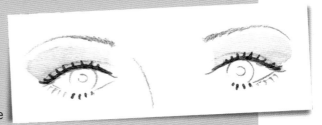

CLOSE-SET EYES

Put extra shadow and liner on the outer corners to draw attention outward. Leave the inner sections and corners clean. Apply one coat of mascara, adding a second coat only to the lashes on the outer edge.

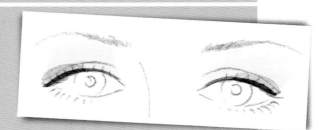

HOODED EYES

Flat lids with no obvious crease—like Asian eyes—can make peepers look smaller. Create the illusion of bigness by simulating a crease's depth. Dust a light shadow all over, then swipe a deeper hue about a quarter of an inch above your lash line.

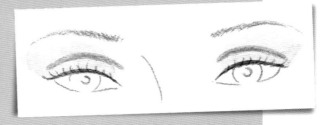

Go for a Smoldering Stare

There's actual scientific proof that guys are total suckers for sultry, smoky eyes. A Massachusetts Institute of Technology study revealed that men are most drawn to a woman when her eyes are shaded darker than the rest of her face. The theory: Across all ethnic groups, women have lighter skin and greater contrast around their eyes than men do. So guys are hardwired to seek out that darkness as a sign of femininity. To create the sexiest eye effect imaginable, reach for soft, shimmery gray shadow hues, which are built to smoke.

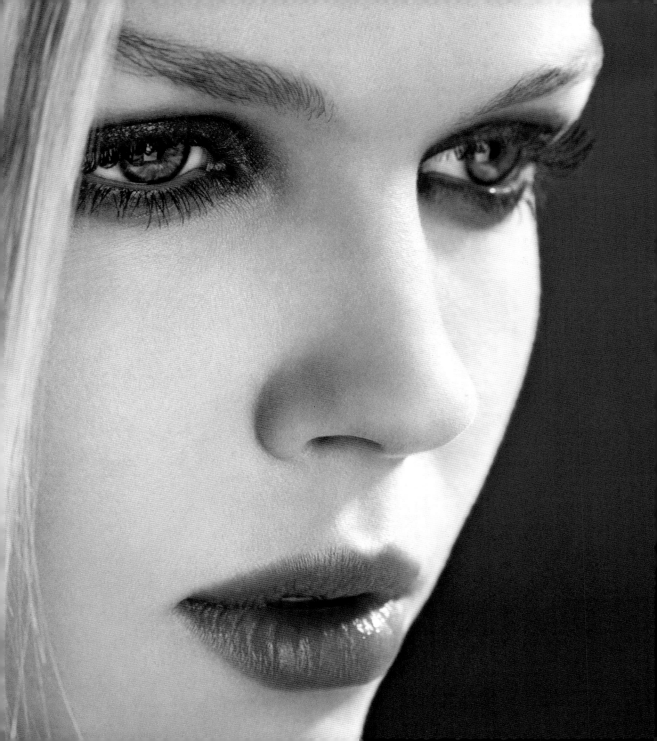

THE BEST LINER LOOKS

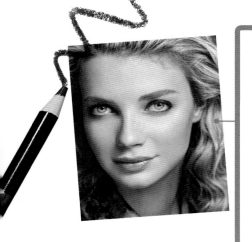

Eyeliner is the MVP of eye makeup—able to make your orbs look sexier in seconds. However, choosing the right formula and color can be tricky. Follow these pointers and your peepers will always look gorge.

■ Daytime Eye Definers

Think subtle colors. Opt for a powder version (it's softer than pencil) in an understated hue like plum, gray, or brown. Your eyes will pop without looking overdone, says NYC makeup artist Laura Geller.

Stay on top. If you prefer pencil to powder, that's also okay during the day, but only draw it on your upper lashes and keep the line superthin. Sharpen your liner first and you'll get a crisp, clean look.

■ P.M. Liner Picks

Try your hand at liquid. You don't need the fine motor skills of a surgeon to master liquid liner. The secret to a perfect application is in the tip: It should be ballpoint pen–size and end in a fine point, says Estée Lauder makeup artist Blair Patterson. Before you paint it on, gently pull your lid taut. Then in one even stroke, glide the liner from the inner eye outward, as close to the lash line as possible. If you're feeling shaky, prop your elbow on a table first.

Go for sparkle. Instead of defining your peepers with a basic black liner for a big night out, go for one that's spiked with flecks of shimmer, says makeup artist Paula Dorf, owner of Paula Dorf Cosmetics. It'll make your eyes look extra-twinkly even in the darkest bar or club. Rim your upper and lower lash lines for extra oomph.

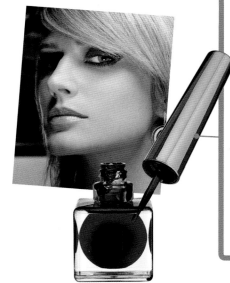

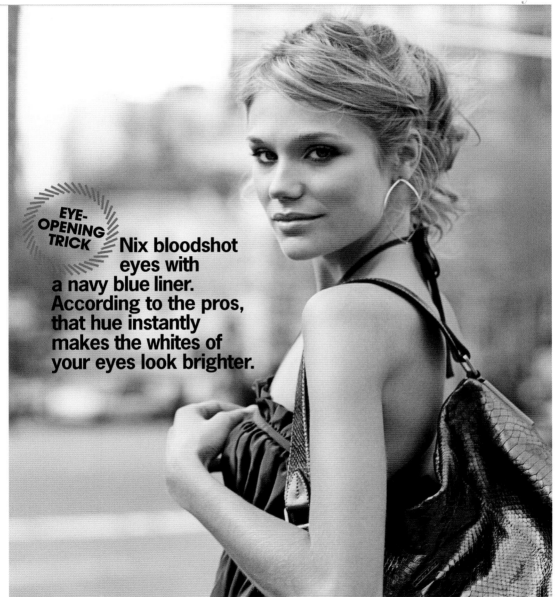

EYE-OPENING TRICK Nix bloodshot eyes with a navy blue liner. According to the pros, that hue instantly makes the whites of your eyes look brighter.

ULTRASEXY LASHES

Moving the wand side-to-side gets mascara on each and every lash.

▓ How to Make Lashes Look...

FATTER
Want superplush lashes that can create a breeze when you blink? Place the mascara brush at the base of your lashes, jiggle it slightly, and pull it through in a slow zigzag motion. This will evenly coat each lash without weighing them down, says makeup artist Jemma Kidd.

LONGER
Curling your lashes is the easiest way to make them look longer. Gently squeeze once at the roots and hold down for five seconds. For major curves, heat your curler with your blow-dryer for a few seconds then let it cool a bit before clamping down.

MORE DENSE
Dot a black or dark brown pencil along your upper lash lines from underneath, says makeup artist Mally Roncal. The key is to get the color right between the lashes.

SEXY SECRET

Coat Your Lower Lashes
Always skip your bottom fringe? Start showing them some love. Swiping your lower lashes with mascara makes your eyes look way bigger, says celeb makeup artist Judy Twine, CEO of Take 5 Cosmetics. Just be sure to hold a tissue under them while stroking the wand to prevent smudges.

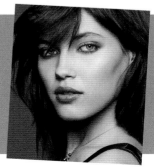

The Lowdown on Fake Fringe

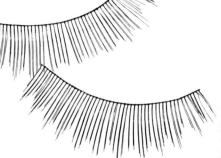

A full, feathery strip of falsies is best for a dramatic evening effect.

Just like hair extensions, fake lashes have become a must-have for celebs. You can get pricey lash extensions, which are glued to your own lashes and last up to a few months, or you can get lush lashes at home. Here's how.

Curl your lashes then squeeze a drop of lash glue onto the back of your hand. Dip a small cluster of lashes (they look more natural than a full strip) into the glue using a tweezer. Next, wedge the end of the lashes between your natural ones at the outer corners of your eyes, using light pressure until they're set. Add a few more, spreading them out evenly along the outer quarter of each eye. Apply mascara to blend the fakes with your real ones.

Fun Fact
Wonder why you often open your mouth when applying mascara? Some of the nerves that open the eyelids are connected to the mouth.
SOURCE: ROBERT CYKIERT, MD, CLINICAL ASSOCIATE PROFESSOR OF OPHTHALMOLOGY AT NYU SCHOOL OF MEDICINE

AMAZING ARCHES

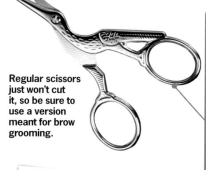

Regular scissors just won't cut it, so be sure to use a version meant for brow grooming.

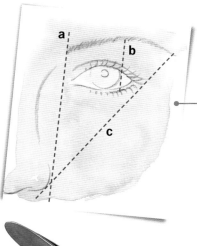

a
b
c

■ How to Shape Your Brows

If you don't want to pay for a pro job, it's okay to go at it on your own. Follow these steps to groom your brows perfectly yourself.

1 **Brush your brows upward**, then use brow scissors to snip just the very ends of any long hairs and repeat brushing downward, says eyebrow pro Ramy Gafni. Trimming the hair before tweezing will reveal the brow shape and remove the weight and bulk so that you can create an ideal shape.

2 **Begin by holding a pencil** parallel to the side of the bridge of your nose (a). The inner edge of your brows should start here. To determine the highest point of your arch, place the pencil parallel to the outside corner of your iris (b). Angling the pencil diagonally from your nostril to the outside corner of your eye will tell you where your brow should end (c). Another foolproof way to locate your arch: "Look at your face straight on in the mirror and find the highest point of your brow. Tweeze directly below it for a perfectly placed arch," says Gafni.

3 **Mark the spots you just mapped out with a brow pencil,** then begin tweezing or waxing accordingly. Remove no more than two rows of hair to maintain a natural effect. You may also need to remove just a few hairs from the top of the outer edges to create a subtle downward slope. If you have thick brows and want a more dramatic arch, remove an additional row from under the peak of the brow to create a more pronounced arch and to keep it from appearing straight and flat.

Brow-Thickening Move

It happens to every chick: You go a little tweezer happy and end up with anorexic arches. To fatten them up, brow groomer Anastasia Soare uses colored brow pomade to fill in sparse areas. The consistency is like hair wax, so it makes brows look thicker while smoothing them.

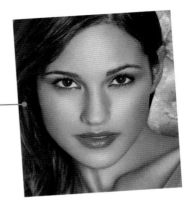

Choose Your Grooming Method

Not sure which arch-shaping option is right for you? Tweezing is best if you don't have a lot of hair to remove or just need to clean up a few strays. Waxing is ideal for naturally bushy or dark brows that grow back quickly. It's also great for cleaning up any fine peach-fuzzy hairs above your brows, says Soare.

How to Find a Pro Plucker
If the arches of the brow person at your salon look great, let her groom yours. Not so much? Ask a friend with a nice set whom she uses.

YOU SHOULD KNOW...

Tinting Your Arches

If you change your hair hue more than two shades, you should alter your brow color too, but only subtly. Arches that match your mane exactly have a tendency to look fake. It's tempting to use dye or bleach, but it's actually illegal (even though some salons do perform the service). You could have an allergic reaction or get it in your eyes, both of which can be dangerous. Instead, use a tinted gel or powder in your desired shade.

COMMON PROBLEMS SOLVED

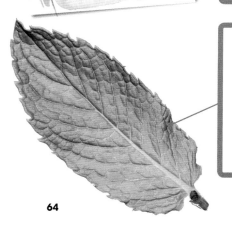

A pale eyeliner can brighten up partied-out eyes.

▨ Get Rid of Redness

It's okay to use whitening eyedrops; just don't overdo it—otherwise, the blood vessels can dilate, causing rebound redness, says NYC ophthalmologist Robert Cykiert. You can also rim the insides of your lower lids with a flesh-toned liner, says New York makeup artist Matin.

▨ Hide Dark Circles

STEP 1: Dab three dots of a concealer that has a peachy-pink tinge to counteract the blue of the circles just under your eyes, from the tear ducts to the outer corners. "Use your ring finger to pat gently and blend it in completely," says makeup artist Mally Roncal. Don't rub—you'll damage the delicate skin there and wipe off the makeup.
STEP 2: Use a clean powder brush to tap a translucent powder lightly over the concealer to set it all day.

▨ Deflate Under-Eye Bags

Gross as it may seem, hemorrhoid cream works on puffy eyes. "Use a tiny bit—just keep it a millimeter from your lashes," says Marguerite McDonald, MD, adjunct clinical professor of ophthalmology at Tulane University Health Sciences Center, in New Orleans. "It will tighten the skin." (Do this only occasionally.) Or try an eye cream with caffeine or mint—both can help shrink dilated blood vessels.

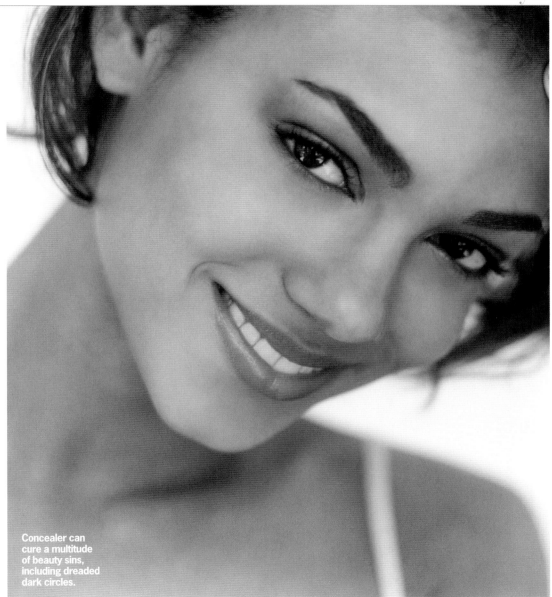

Concealer can cure a multitude of beauty sins, including dreaded dark circles.

Lips

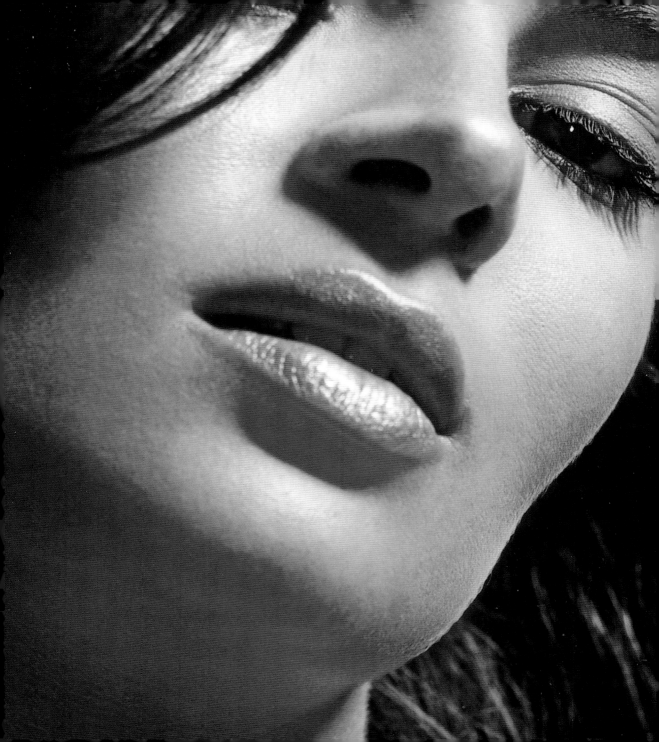

SECRETS OF

Alluring Lips

■ Nothing says "Kiss me now" more than an enticing mouth. And there are three key qualities that separate an ordinary smacker from one that men just can't keep their lips off: a plush, pillowlike appearance, a smooth-as-satin surface, and an inviting, juicy hue. Don't worry if you weren't born with a plus-size pout since we'll tell you how to fake it, plus we have many more moves to make your mouth its most desirable.

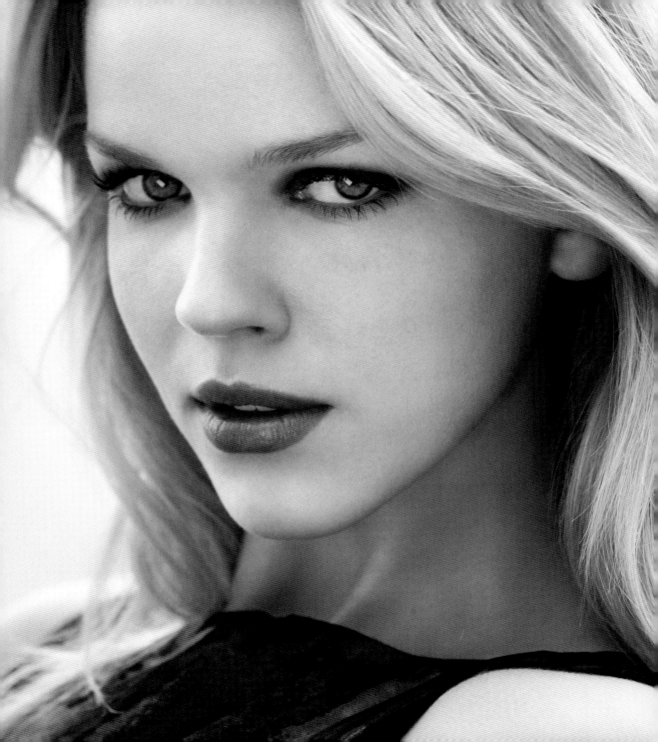

THE BEGINNINGS OF
A BEAUTIFUL MOUTH

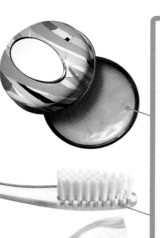

The most enticing lips are full, soft, and naturally rosy. To prime your kisser for lip color (and smooching), follow these steps:

1 Swipe on some lip balm, then use your fingertips to massage it in. Its conditioning agents will fill cracks on chapped lips, says New York makeup artist Susan Giordano. Work it in for 30 seconds or so—this helps stimulate blood vessels and ensures that your lips look their absolute fullest.

2 Next, run a dry extrasoft toothbrush or wet washcloth over your mouth to slough off dead skin cells. (Hot tip: Do it in the shower—the steam will soften those yucky dry bits so that they fall right off.) You also can polish on the go with a pinch of sugar. It melts quickly, so it won't irritate delicate skin.

3 Finish by blotting lips with a tissue to soak up a leftover residue. Still a tad dry? Dab on a bit of nongreasy lip balm.

YOU SHOULD KNOW...
Protect Your Pout
The thin skin on your lips is vulnerable to the sun year-round. Prevent rays from parching your pucker by applying a balm or gloss that contains SPF 15 during the day.

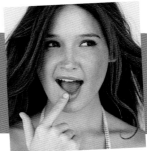

Pampering Treat

Whip up this special homemade lip mask from skin-care expert Cornelia Zicu when your pout requires a little extra attention. Mix three teaspoons of petroleum jelly with one teaspoon of honey and a dash of cinnamon. Store the concoction in an empty lip-balm pot and massage it on at night using smooth, slow strokes. Leave on for 30 minutes before wiping off. Your lips will feel velvety smooth.

INSTANT LIP-PLUMPING MOVES

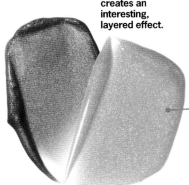

Double impact: Using two glosses creates an interesting, layered effect.

- Don't half-ass it when it comes to applying your favorite lip plumpers (i.e., products that use hyaluronic acid or mild irritants to temporarily swell lip tissue). Slather the stuff on! Just make sure your lips are totally naked. Any moisture—either from saliva or a balm—will prevent the formula from penetrating.

- Use two complementary lip hues. Swipe on a shimmery rose-colored gloss, then apply a paler pink version over it, says makeup artist Carol Shaw. Layering two colors creates the illusion of depth so your mouth looks ultraplush.

How to Fake a Fuller Mouth With Makeup

Celebrity makeup artist Mally Roncal breaks it down.

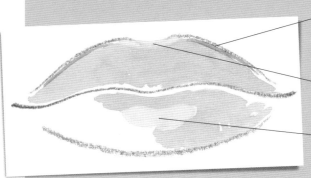

LINER. Line lips with a pencil that matches your lips, then smudge the color over the ridge of your pout with your finger. But skip the corners of your mouth—it can visually close in your lips.

HIGHLIGHTER. Blend a thin line of liquid highlighter along your cupid's bow so light will bounce off it and play up this curvy area.

GLOSS. Swipe on a neutral lip color, then place a dab of shimmery gloss on the center of your bottom lip. This will reflect light for a bee-stung effect.

● You can whip up your own plumping product at home. Celebrity skin guru Sonya Dakar swears by her technique—mixing a teaspoon of regular olive oil with a pinch of salt then dabbing it on your mouth. "These are the key ingredients in my lip balm," she reveals. "The oil is very moisturizing, and the sodium makes the thin skin on your lips puff up fast."

● When you're in the market for a new lip gloss, the key is to go for the absolute shiniest, most shimmer-infused one you can find (look for words that suggest moisture, like *wet*, *juicy*, or *slick*). The reason? The more reflective the formula, the fuller it will make your lips look.

● In general, when you want to fatten up your lips, stick with hydrating lip products, such as glosses and creamy lipsticks. They contain moisturizing ingredients like emollients, vitamin E, and shea butter, which give your mouth a plusher payoff than drier lip stains and matte formulas.

● After applying a dark lipstick shade (which can be minimizing), dab a small makeup brush in a concealer that's slightly lighter than your foundation, then run the brush along the outskirts of your lip line. "The contrast between your lipstick and the surrounding lightness will make your entire mouth appear larger," says makeup artist and cosmetics creator Vincent Longo.

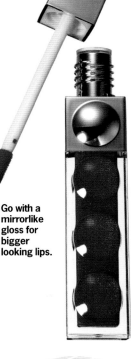

Go with a mirrorlike gloss for bigger looking lips.

Smacker Stamina
Lip plumpers typically work for only four to five hours, so bring yours with you when you're going out.

Seduction Secret

A surefire way to get his attention: Apply lipstick in front of him. "When a woman purses her lips, it makes her look more provocative and, therefore, more desirable," says Michael Cunningham, PhD, a psychologist in the department of communication at the University of Louisville. But you've got to get into it. "If she looks like she likes the feeling of her lips against the lipstick, it signals on a subconscious level that she's eager to be kissed," says relationship expert Scott Kudia, PhD.

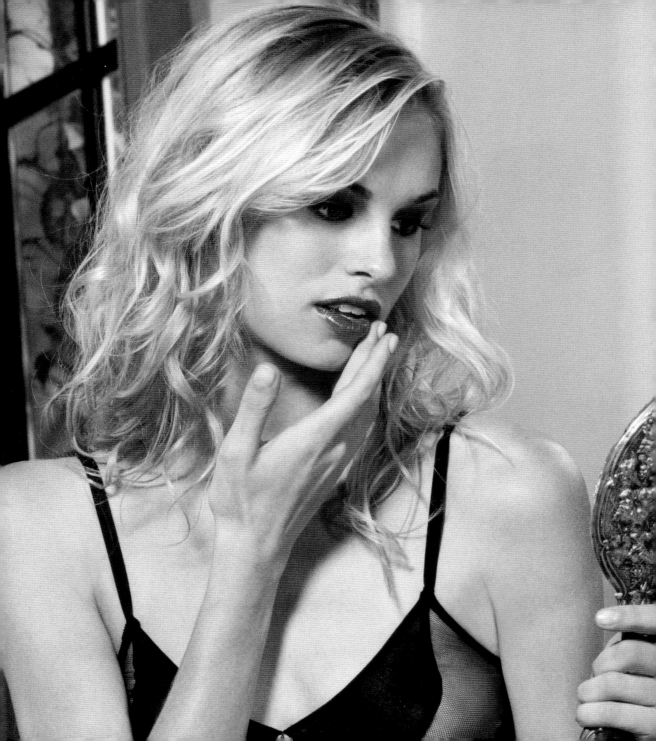

APPLY YOUR LIP COLOR LIKE A PRO

Prime your lips with foundation before applying a pale lip hue.

■ Get the Exact Color You See in the Tube

Lightly dot your lips with foundation before applying a nude or flesh-toned lipstick. Creating this neutral base will ensure that the color looks the same on your kisser as it does in the tube.

■ Loosen Up Your Lips

For a flawless lip color application, let your mouth go a bit slack. If you pucker up or tense it, you won't get an even finish.

■ Postapplication Trick

To prevent your lipstick from migrating onto your teeth, (never an attractive thing), close your lips around your pointer finger then pull it out to remove any excess color from your inner lips.

YOU SHOULD KNOW...

Try Before You Buy

It's so tempting to use the lipstick testers at a store, but just think about the germs on those things—gross! Here's a safe technique: Scrape the top of the bullet with a cotton swab, then scoop off a bit of color and apply with a fresh swab.

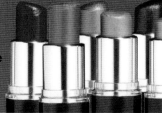

Make Teeth Look Brighter

If you want more brilliant looking chompers, you have two options—go to a pro or do it yourself. An in-office version will whiten your teeth about eight to nine shades (think the subtle difference between colors on a paint strip). An at-home kit will give you about a four-shade improvement.

Regardless of the method, know that your pearly whites can only get so bright, no matter how many times you bleach them, so any treatments you do after reaching your maximum level of whiteness (they shouldn't be whiter than the whites of your eyes) are more hurtful than helpful, says Cyrus Tahmasebi, a dentist with BriteSmile.

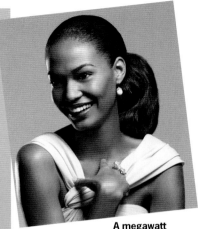

A megawatt smile is supersexy.

Instant Smile Fixer
A lipstick or gloss with blue undertones, such as plum or cherry, will downplay any yellowness in your enamel so your teeth look whiter.

PUT YOUR COLOR ON LOCKDOWN

■ Start With a Primer

Vibrant lip hues can go on sizzling then start fizzling before you're done with your first cocktail. Use a lip primer (it's like a base coat for your mouth) and the color will stay fresh for hours.

■ Line Your Whole Mouth

Make any gloss or lipstick last longer by first filling in your entire mouth with a matching lip liner. When the top layer fades, the liner will still be there but not in an unattractive ring-around-the-mouth way.

Liner acts like border patrol for your lip color.

■ Use Invisible Lip Liner

If traditional lip liner just isn't your thing, try a clear version. Trace the outer edges of your mouth after you apply lipstick. The waxy texture will keep color pigments in place.

SEXY SECRET
Smooch-Proof Your Pout

For a sexy lip look that can withstand a steamy make-out session, dab a rosy lip stain onto your mouth. These formulas are like indelible ink and won't budge until you take them off...and even then you're gonna have to scrub!

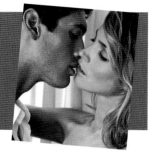

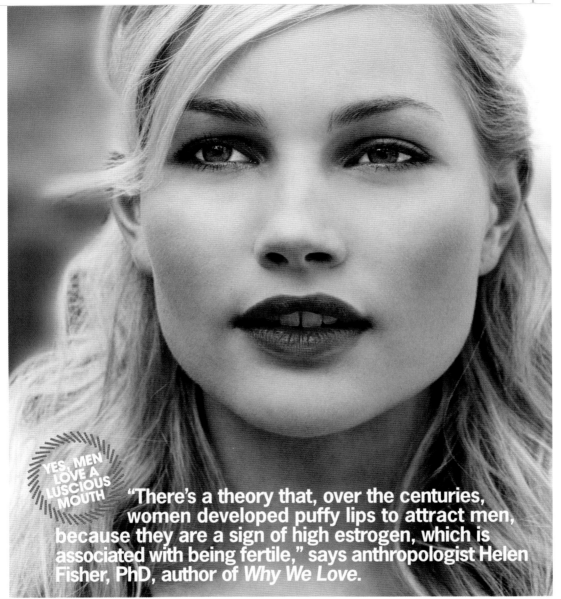

YES, MEN LOVE A LUSCIOUS MOUTH

"There's a theory that, over the centuries, women developed puffy lips to attract men, because they are a sign of high estrogen, which is associated with being fertile," says anthropologist Helen Fisher, PhD, author of *Why We Love*.

THE SEXY MESSAGE
A SCARLET MOUTH SENDS

A red is a red is a red, right? Wrong. Leatrice Eiseman, author of *More Alive With Color*, decodes what the most sizzling versions of this hue convey.

PEACH RED The gold and fire tones are for women who enjoy life at full throttle.

ROSE This stimulating shade energizes the wearer and those looking at her.

WINE The complex blend appeals to those who like to cause a stir.

BLACK CHERRY Its dark and seductive effect makes it the ultimate power color.

WHAT IT SAYS TO THE WORLD

"I'm bubbly, approachable, and always out to have a good time."

"Pay attention to me. I know I'm sexy, and you should too."

"I'm sensual and mysterious. I don't need to broadcast what I'm thinking."

"I am elegant and sophisticated and love a challenge."

YOU SHOULD KNOW...

Dark Lipstick Hint

When you're sporting a rich-colored lipstick, it's best to apply it straight from the tube. "Using your fingers or even a lip brush will make the color too sheer," says NYC makeup artist Mathew Nigara. Start at the middle of your lips, and work the color to the outer edges. Stay away from the corners—the color will seep there on its own.

Why Red Lips Drive Guys Crazy

You already know that the color red is associated with love and passion, but get this: Studies show that when people look at a crimson hue, their pulses and respiration rates speed up. "Red is energetic and sends the message that you are sexy and exciting," says Lisa Herbert, executive vice president of the fashion, home, and consumer division at Pantone, a company that specializes in color.

Bottom line: There's no better hue to wear on your lips to make your date's heart race—literally.

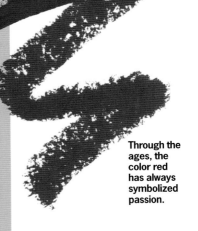

Through the ages, the color red has always symbolized passion.

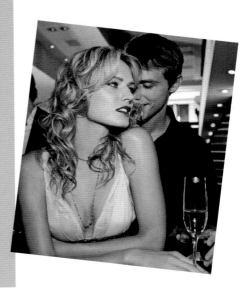

HOT LIP LOOKS
TO TRY TONIGHT

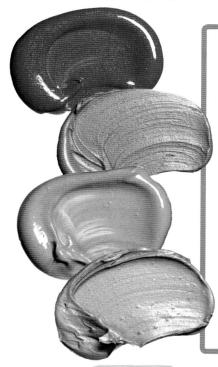

4 Come-Hither Shades

These juicy lip colors are vibrant but not overbearing. Plus, they look sexy as hell on everyone.

■ Shiny Cherry Red
Go for a true red without yellow or blue undertones.

■ Pinched-Cheek Pink
A pink hue with a hint of red is one notch brighter than a naturally flushed look…and flushed spells flirty.

■ Shimmery Gold Coral
Tangerine tints look most alluring with hints of gold iridescence.

■ Naughty Mauvey Nude
Pick a flesh-toned lipstick with a hint of mauve—otherwise the hue could look washed out.

SEXY SECRET
Get a Lusty Lip Effect

For "kiss me" lips, apply a creamy lipstick in a hue that is one shade darker than the fleshy inside of your lip, advises makeup artist Mally Roncal. It shouldn't look too precise, so leave the lip liner behind…and don't worry about applying it perfectly.

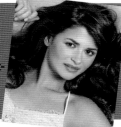

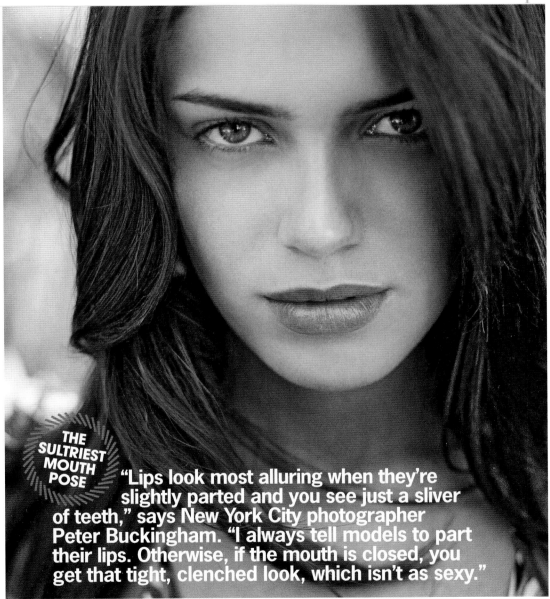

THE SULTRIEST MOUTH POSE "Lips look most alluring when they're slightly parted and you see just a sliver of teeth," says New York City photographer Peter Buckingham. "I always tell models to part their lips. Otherwise, if the mouth is closed, you get that tight, clenched look, which isn't as sexy."

Hair

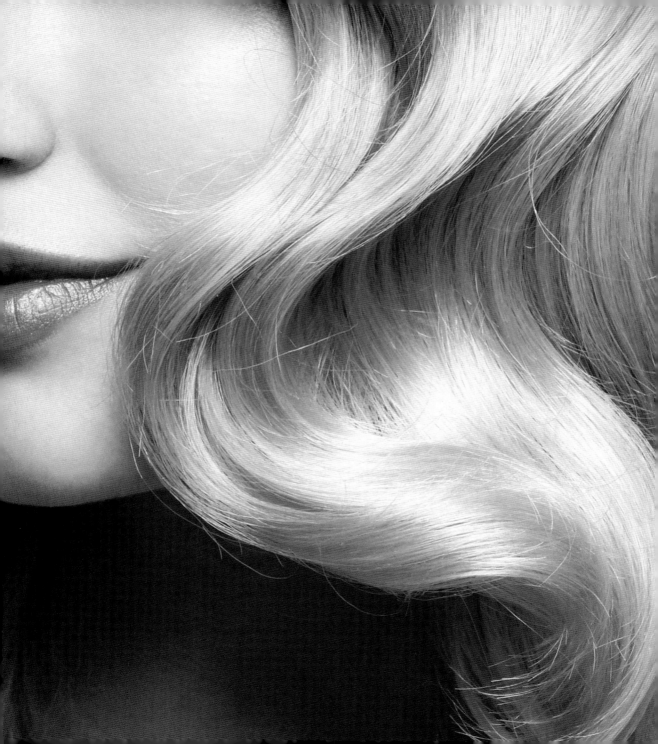

Amazing Hair

All the beauty energy you expend tending to your tresses is well worth it, since few things are as eye-catching as a gorgeous head of hair.

In this section you'll learn how to get every aspect of sexy, healthy strands: shine, softness, movement, and volume. There's also advice on dealing with a slew of common hair traumas, plus tips on how to determine the perfect hair color for you. And of course, Cosmo will turn you on to the hottest hairstyles on the planet. The mane you've always wanted is just a few pages away.

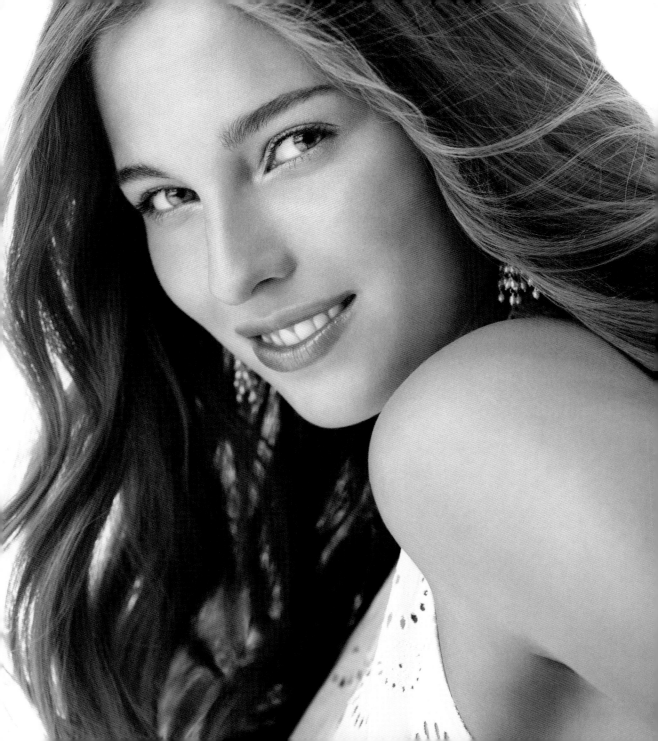

HEALTHY HAIR STRATEGIES

Split Ends Rx
A temporary fix for tattered tips: Apply shine serum to damp ends then blow-dry them using a paddle brush while aiming the nozzle downward.

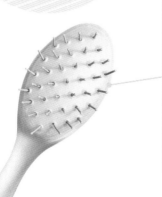

Getting hot locks can be a catch-22: You assault your mane with blow-dryers, brushes, and styling tools to make it look great. But over time, all that primping can leave hair dull and brittle. What's a girl to do? Follow our advice for preventing tress distress.

Suds up less often. Wash your mane every two days with a gentle shampoo to avoid stripping it of its natural oils.

Condition with care. Daily wear and tear saps hair of moisture. In addition to using a regular conditioner, treat your locks (especially your ends, which are driest) to a weekly intensive mask.

Keep tools in top shape. Old, worn bristles on your brush can rough up your hair's cuticle. When shopping for a new one, run it down your arm. If the bristles feel abrasive, skip it. And while you already know that it's best to detangle wet strands with a wide-tooth comb, African-American babes should do it in the shower, right after applying conditioner, to protect your fragile tresses.

YOU SHOULD KNOW...
Scrub Your Scalp

A head massage not only feels amazing, but all that rubbing removes product buildup and boosts circulation so more nutrients can get to the hair follicle. So beg your stylist for an extra-long scrub session or do it yourself at home using your fingertips.

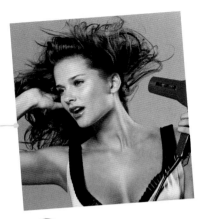

Blow-dry, don't blowtorch, your hair. Before you even as much as look at your blow-dryer, apply a thermal protective styling product (pick one that calls this out on the bottle). Dry your locks at least 50 percent with your dryer on the low-heat setting. Then you can crank up the heat and wield a brush. Once you get going, hold the dryer 3 inches away from your hair, point it downward, and keep it in constant motion to prevent fried sections.

Move on from metal. Go for a ceramic flatiron or curling iron. Unlike metal models, ceramic heats up evenly, so there are no strand-scorching hot spots. Another rule of thumb: Don't heat any one section of hair longer than three counts of "Mississippi."

TLC for African-American Strands

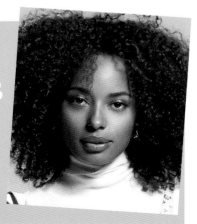

Blot, don't rub, damp hair when you get out of the shower and always apply a leave-in conditioner when styling your hair with heat. Also, when you're using a blow-dryer, keep it on the lowest setting the whole time.

SHINY HAIR HINTS

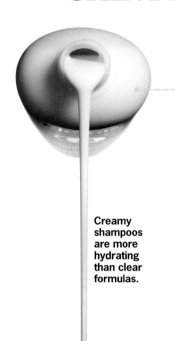

Creamy shampoos are more hydrating than clear formulas.

A gleaming mane ensures that all eyes are on you, which is what you want, isn't it? Follow these tips to get luscious locks.

- Start with a moisturizing shampoo and conditioner. Look for hydrating ingredients, such as olive oil, shea butter, and dimethicone, says Mark DeVincenzo, creative director of Frédéric Fekkai salon in NYC.

- Use the right shine-enhancing product for your strand type. If you have thick or coarse hair, apply a silicone-based serum or a styling cream to wet hair, then add another coat when strands are dry. If your mane is medium-textured, hit the bottom few inches with a shine spray after blow-drying. And if you have fine locks, mist your palms with an extra-light shine spray then run it just over your ends, says DeVincenzo.

- Try an at-home clear gloss treatment, which will infuse your strands with potent polishers like silicone, jojoba oil, and vitamin E. Follow the directions on the packaging carefully. The mirrorlike luster will last for a week or more.

SEXY SECRET

Major Mane Booster

Chopsticks have a hidden use: They can give your hair loads of volume. Right after blow-drying, while your hair is still warm, twist it into a bun and slip the sticks through, says NYC salon owner Ted Gibson. Remove the sticks when your tresses have cooled and voilà—beautiful body.

Bigger Is Better—
How to Get Tons of Volume

Cosmo's covers are famous for featuring women with voluminous, bombshell hair. Here, Oscar Blandi, who's styled many Cosmo covers, explains how to get our signature strand effect.

1. Towel dry your hair then mist a leave-in conditioner on your ends followed by a volumizer all over. Flip your head over and start blow-drying your roots while pulling them away from your scalp with your fingers, then dry the rest of your hair until it's slightly damp.

2. Bring your hair upright and wrap 1-inch sections in Velcro rollers. Once all your hair is set, blow-dry with a diffuser for 10 minutes on the hot setting, then 10 minutes on cool. Alternative options: Use large hot rollers or a curling iron but first make sure hair is 100 percent dry.

3. Remove the rollers, then mix a drop each of shine serum and light gel (the perfect combo for hold and shine) between your fingers, then run hands throughout your hair.

4. For an extra body boost, gently tease your roots around the crown of your head, Finish by finger-tousling your hair into a cascade of loose come-hither curls, and give your locks a light spritz with hair spray.

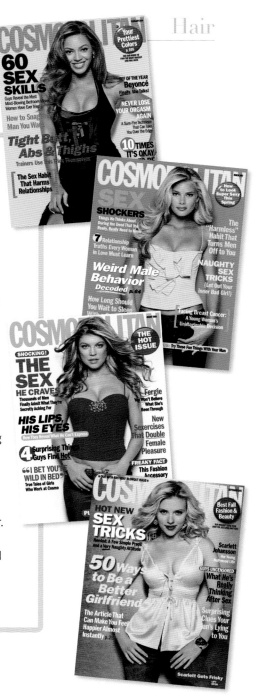

THE PERFECT BLOWOUT...
YOU CAN DO YOURSELF

Certain hairstyles come and go but swingy, smooth, polished strands always look hot. Here, Redken creative consultant Guido shares his strategy for giving yourself a pro blowout.

1 Run a dollop of smoothing cream through damp locks, then use jaw clips to separate your hair into four to six sections. Decide now if you want to make a center or a side part and arrange accordingly. Start blow-drying at the area closest to your neck.

2 Stylists use a rolling round brush technique to create ultrasmooth results. Here's how to do it: Grab a 2-inch section of hair then nestle a large round brush into the roots; the bristles should go deep inside the hair. Pull the brush all the way down the hair shaft, but don't let the ends fall off since you need the tension to straighten your hair. Roll the brush back up and repeat a few times. Keep the blow-dryer pointed in a downward position while your wrist continuously rolls the brush up and down the hair shaft. It should take three passes or so to dry each section.

3 Once your hair is totally dry, go back over just your hairline once more to tame any kinks. You can use a flatiron, but avoid your roots since you don't want them to be too flat.

4 Mist your palms with shine spray and run them lightly over your hair, concentrating at the ends.

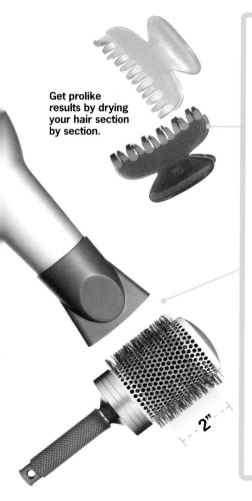

Get prolike results by drying your hair section by section.

2"

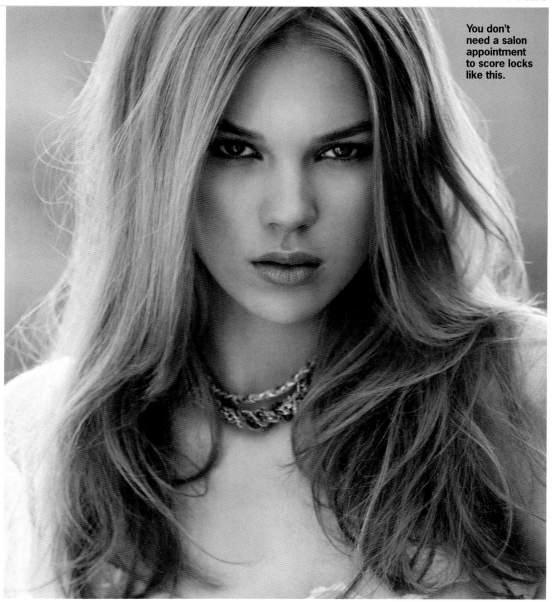

You don't
need a salon
appointment
to score locks
like this.

FOXY HAIR—IN A FLASH

Just because you don't have tons of primping time doesn't mean you can't look hot.

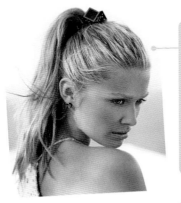

■ Whip Up a Posh Ponytail

What upgrades your usual fallback style from simple to sexy? Location, location, location. Perch it at the crown of your head, and it won't channel a cheerleader. To do it, flip your head upside down to position the pony as high as possible, and secure it with a chic elastic for extra polish. Back-comb the top inch of the tail to add some oomph at the roots.

A deep side part creates a simple but sophisticated style.

■ Flip Your Part

One of the fastest styles you can create without a pair of scissors? A low side part. It's so dramatic and instantly chic, plus, it's great for all hair types and textures. All you have to do is part hair about 4 to 6 inches above the ear then sweep strands back with one of the teeth on your comb. Smooth any flyaways with a drop of shine serum.

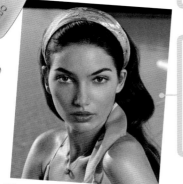

■ Don Something Dazzling

If you're running crazy late for a party and your hair is only semi-done, slip on a flashy headband or a silk scarf. It makes such a glamorous statement, without any hassle. For maximum effect, pick something that has a colorful, eye-catching print.

Cosmo's Sexiest Beauty Secrets

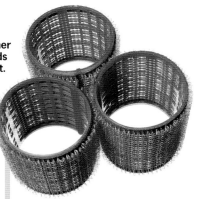

The larger the rollers, the smoother your strands will turn out.

Revive a Day-Old Blowout

If you don't have an hour to wash and blow out your hair, fake a fresh style fast by using three big Velcro rollers on just your face-framing strands. Put one at the top of your hairline and one at each temple. Mist them with hair spray to help dry up any oil and set the hair in place. Blast the rollers with your hair dryer, then leave them in for five minutes. The end result: a style that looks like you just slaved over it.

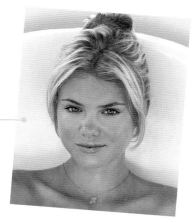

Do the Lazy Updo

Fast-track an updo by teasing the hair around the crown of your head with a fine-tooth comb then giving it a shot of hair spray. Next, brush the hair to smooth it out a bit and pull everything back into a high, loose bun, allowing a few pieces to fall around your face.

Revive Your Roots in Record Time

When you need to oomph up flat hair on the double, rub a tiny dab of a lightweight sculpting wax between your palms until you just see a bit of sheen on your hands, then scrunch up your roots. You'll bulk up fine hair without weighing it down if you stick with a light water-based version.

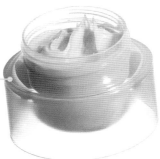

SURVIVE ANY
HAIR DISASTER

Having a heinous hair moment before a date or botched an at-home dye job? Fear not...Cosmo's coming to the rescue with EMT (Emergency Mane Treatment) advice.

How to Recover From Hat Hair

Sure, hats are cool to wear, but their evil spawn—hat hair—is anything but sexy. Here's what you can do to help prevent it.

STEP 1: First, nix static (which gives you a ton of flyaways) by running a fabric-softener sheet over your hair or misting your brush with Static Guard before running it through your strands root-to-tip.

STEP 2: Now, fluff it up. Lift matted-down roots by flipping your head upside down and gently massaging them to boost volume.

How to Fix a Dud Dye Job

Orange roots are a telltale sign of a bad at-home hair color experience. How to deal:

STEP 1: See a colorist as soon as possible. If you try to fix the problem on your own, you'll just make it worse. This process is typically more complicated than a straight coloring job, so be prepared to pay a bit more than usual for what the pros call color correction.

STEP 2: Until your appointment, wear your hair curly or tousled to make your color appear more blended.

How to Disguise a Bad Home Bang Trim

You thought you were so savvy trimming your own fringe—until you chopped off an inch where a centimeter would've sufficed. Here, some possible remedies to hide your mistakes until they grow back.

OPTION 1: Part your hair on the side where your bangs are the longest, then sweep them across your forehead so they fall over the too-short bits. Bonus: Side-swept bangs are flattering on all face shapes.

OPTION 2: The more piecey your do looks, the more effectively your unsightly bangs will be camouflaged. Work a dab of pomade between your fingertips, then twirl little sections of hair from roots to ends.

OPTION 3: If your bangs are too short but not crooked, brush them against your forehead and place a thick scarf or headband at your hairline to nudge them down to a normal-looking length.

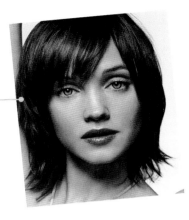

A dusting of powder can cure a case of the greasies.

How to Deal With Product Overload

If you overestimated the amount of goo to use and now your strands look really dull or oil-slicked, take these measures depending on the type of styler you OD'd on.

PROBLEM 1: Hair spray, mousse, and gel: Brush, brush, brush. Let your bristles revive your locks for you. These products are alcohol-based (and therefore dry), so they comb right out.

PROBLEM 2: Shine serum and smoothing cream: Sprinkle on a shake of talcum powder to absorb the grease, then finger-style.

PROBLEM 3: Pomade, wax, paste, and thick balms: Spritz alcohol-based hair spray over the gunky parts. It will help dry up some of the gook. Then gently use a comb to separate any sticky strands.

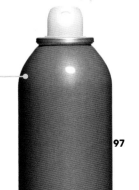

FIND YOUR PERFECT HAIR HUE

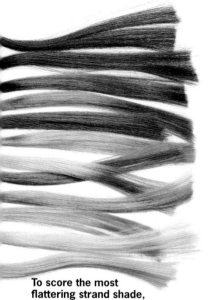

To score the most flattering strand shade, use your eyebrow color as a guide.

While it's fun to experiment with a range of tress tints, at some point you'll want to settle on a shade that works wonders for you. These hints will help you devise a foolproof strategy.

- **Rule of thumb:** Pick a base color that's no more than two shades lighter or darker than your eyebrows.

- **Why it works:** The brow color you're born with complements your skin tone perfectly. Stray too far from it and your complexion will appear washed out. (Dyeing your brows won't make a difference—the benchmark is always their natural color.) You can also use your true base shade as a barometer. But if you can't remember it exactly (or don't have pictures of yourself at age 12 handy), you're better off going by your brows.

- **Also keep in mind:** Weaving blond highlights into your base color enhances any complexion. Like self-tanner, golden tones illuminate your skin. Keep the streaks thin to ensure everything blends in well.

SOURCE: LOGICS COLORIST JENNIFER J.

YOU SHOULD KNOW...

The Best Blond for Dark Skin

These days, lots of dark-skinned chicks are making a major mane statement by going blond—think Beyoncé, Tyra Banks, and Mary J. Blige. "The contrast between dark skin and light hair can be really striking, but it's tricky to do yourself," says stylist Kim Kimble. "A pro will know the right shade for your skin tone." The basics: Women with deep brown skin should go with a rich honey hue. If your complexion is a medium tone, try a sandy color. And if you have lighter skin, you can pull off a pale golden blond. To keep strands healthy, do a deep-conditioning treatment at home twice a week, especially if you also relax your hair, says celebrity colorist Rita Hazan.

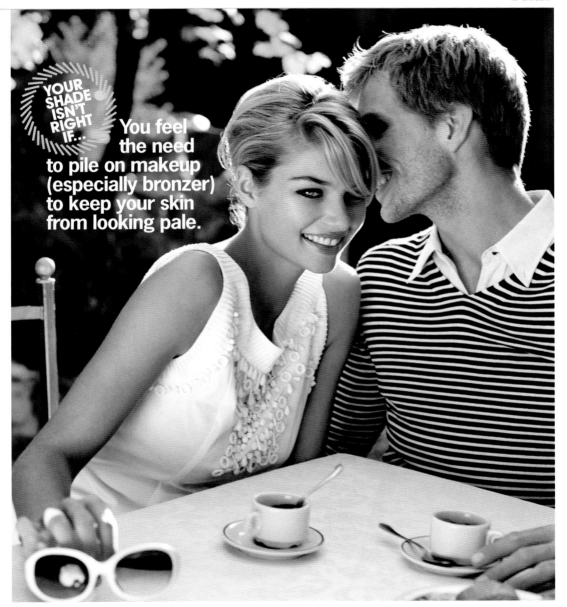

YOUR SHADE ISN'T RIGHT IF... You feel the need to pile on makeup (especially bronzer) to keep your skin from looking pale.

PULL OFF A PRO DYE JOB AT HOME

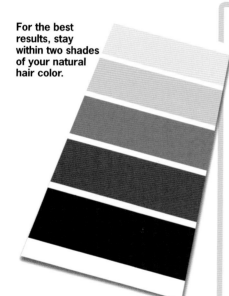

For the best results, stay within two shades of your natural hair color.

Time It Right
Start your timer as soon as you begin applying the formula and don't leave anything on for more than 30 minutes or you'll cook your hair, warns celebrity colorist Rita Hazan.

It's easier than ever to tint your own tresses since today's hair-color kits are very sophisticated. But there are a few tips you won't find on the back of the box that will help you get gorgeous results.

● **When you're going darker,** use a semipermanent formula the first time around. If you like the shade, wait until it fades and then apply a permanent version. Start in the back and save the strands around your face for last. The front pieces of your hair tend to be porous (due to daily wear and tear), so they'll absorb more color than the back and underside.

● **When you're lightening up,** look for a permanent shade that has the words *neutral, beige,* or *ash* in the name to prevent your hair from looking brassy. Start in the front and work your way to the back so the pieces around your face are the brightest. If you want to go even lighter, you can use a highlighting kit afterward. Warning: Dark brown hair can sometimes turn orangey if you lift it more than two levels, so go to a pro if your natural base is darker than a medium brown.

● **When you're touching up your roots,** whether you've lightened or darkened your hair, you should apply color to the regrowth only (the part closest to your scalp) so you don't overprocess your locks or end up with an uneven hue.

SOURCE: MARIE ROBINSON, SENIOR COLORIST
AT SALLY HERSHBERGER DOWNTOWN SALON, IN NYC

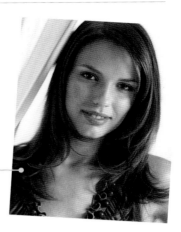

■ Protect and Preserve Your Hue

Investing your time and money in a new hue is only worth it if it lasts, which means you'll get more out of the shade if you treat it right.

● Avoid washing your hair for about 24 hours after coloring it. When it's time to lather up, opt for a color-safe shampoo and conditioner that contain UV protection, and steer clear of clarifying or deep cleansing formulas, which can strip dye pigments. And in general, avoid shampooing every day to prevent fading.

● Gloss treatments enrich your natural color without depositing any dye. Try an at-home version or treat yourself to the salon experience. Most take only a few minutes to activate, so you'll pay less than you would for a full head of highlights or a single-process color.

SOURCE: ROBBIE CONTRERAS, COLOR DIRECTOR
AT TELA HAIR SALON IN NYC

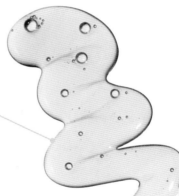

SEXY SECRET

Go Streaking

The trick to getting hot highlights is all in where you place them. You'd never get ruler-straight, evenly spaced streaks naturally from the sun, so don't layer them on that way. At home, keep highlights between ⅛- and ¼-inch thick, and don't overlook the hairline, since those pieces will brighten your face.

15 Hot, Hot Hairstyles

Craving a fresh look? Get inspired by these lock options. Whether your hair is long or short, curly or straight (or in-between), there's a do here for you, plus tips on how to get it and an easy way to switch it up. So what are you waiting for? Go find your sexy new style!

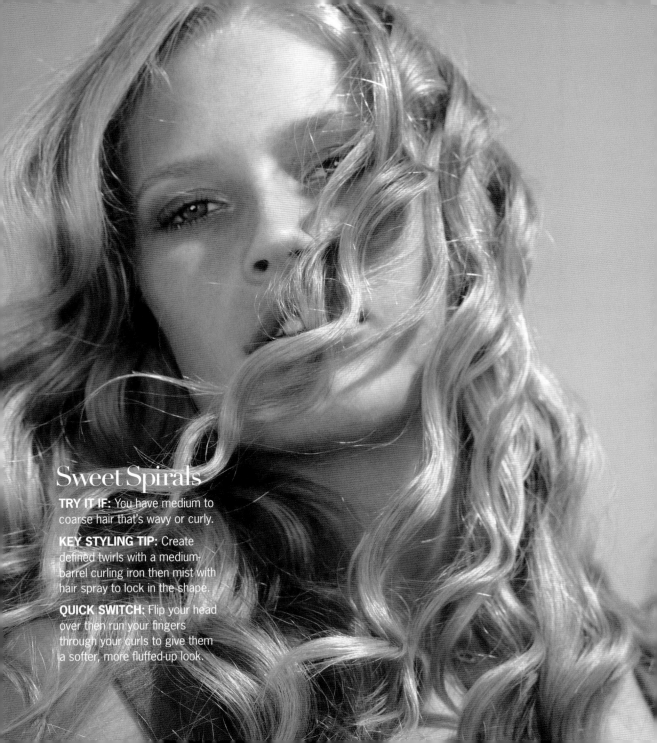

Sweet Spirals

TRY IT IF: You have medium to coarse hair that's wavy or curly.

KEY STYLING TIP: Create defined twirls with a medium-barrel curling iron then mist with hair spray to lock in the shape.

QUICK SWITCH: Flip your head over then run your fingers through your curls to give them a softer, more fluffed-up look.

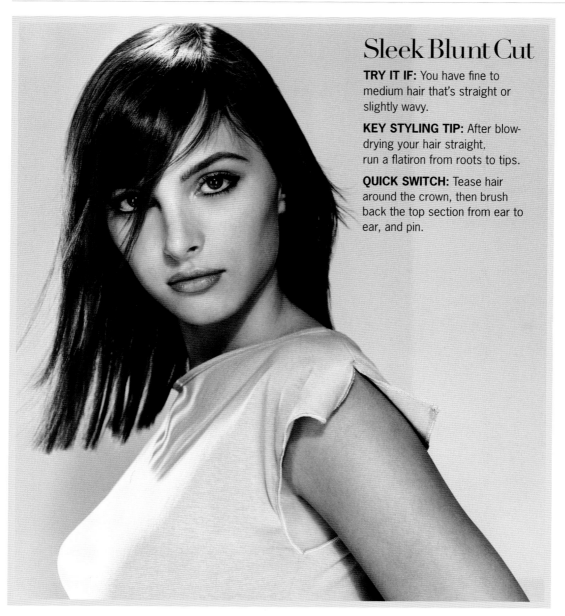

Sleek Blunt Cut

TRY IT IF: You have fine to medium hair that's straight or slightly wavy.

KEY STYLING TIP: After blow-drying your hair straight, run a flatiron from roots to tips.

QUICK SWITCH: Tease hair around the crown, then brush back the top section from ear to ear, and pin.

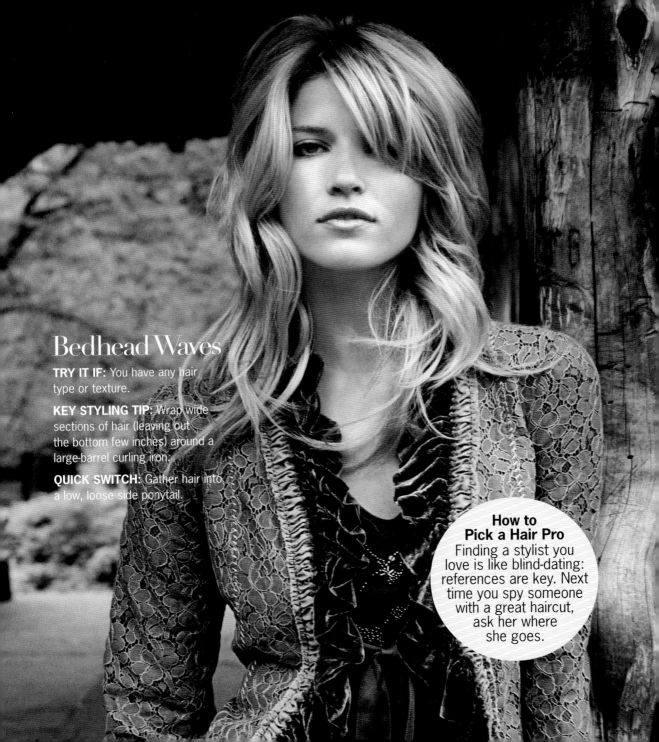

Bedhead Waves

TRY IT IF: You have any hair type or texture.

KEY STYLING TIP: Wrap wide sections of hair (leaving out the bottom few inches) around a large-barrel curling iron.

QUICK SWITCH: Gather hair into a low, loose side ponytail.

How to Pick a Hair Pro
Finding a stylist you love is like blind-dating: references are key. Next time you spy someone with a great haircut, ask her where she goes.

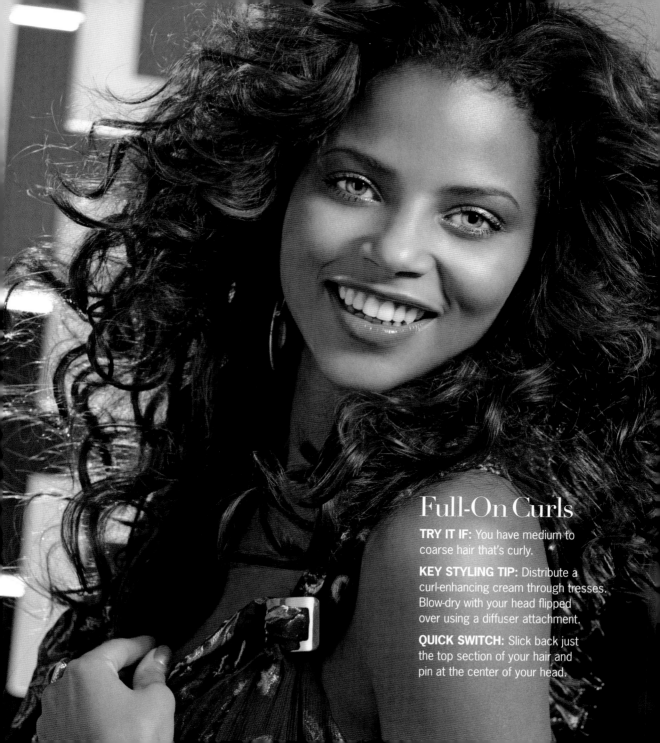

Full-On Curls

TRY IT IF: You have medium to coarse hair that's curly.

KEY STYLING TIP: Distribute a curl-enhancing cream through tresses. Blow-dry with your head flipped over using a diffuser attachment.

QUICK SWITCH: Slick back just the top section of your hair and pin at the center of your head.

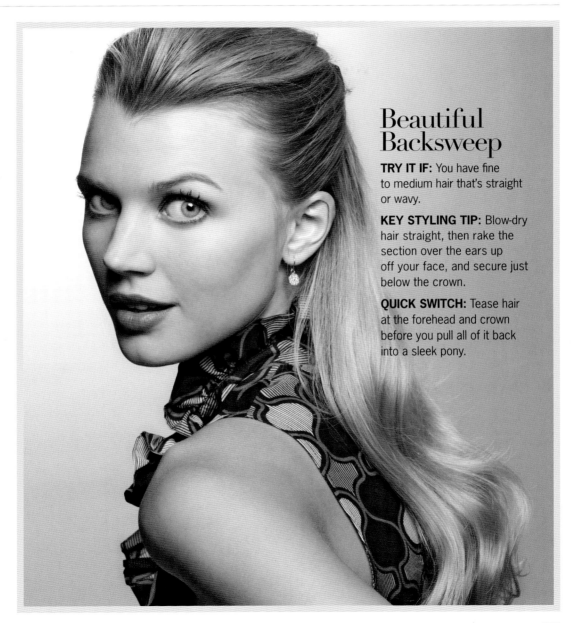

Beautiful Backsweep

TRY IT IF: You have fine to medium hair that's straight or wavy.

KEY STYLING TIP: Blow-dry hair straight, then rake the section over the ears up off your face, and secure just below the crown.

QUICK SWITCH: Tease hair at the forehead and crown before you pull all of it back into a sleek pony.

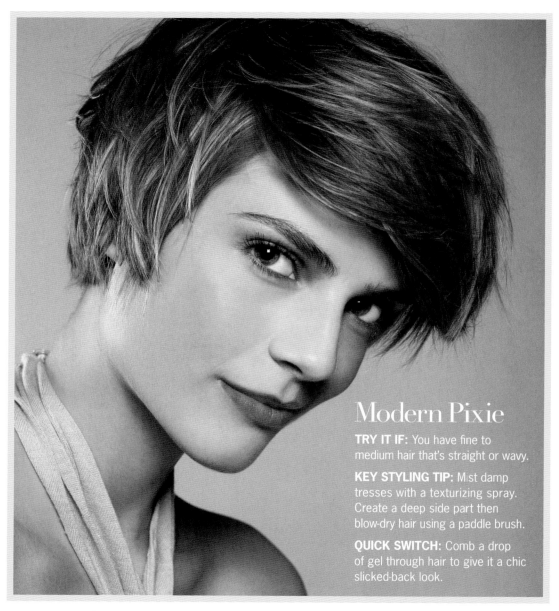

Modern Pixie

TRY IT IF: You have fine to medium hair that's straight or wavy.

KEY STYLING TIP: Mist damp tresses with a texturizing spray. Create a deep side part then blow-dry hair using a paddle brush.

QUICK SWITCH: Comb a drop of gel through hair to give it a chic slicked-back look.

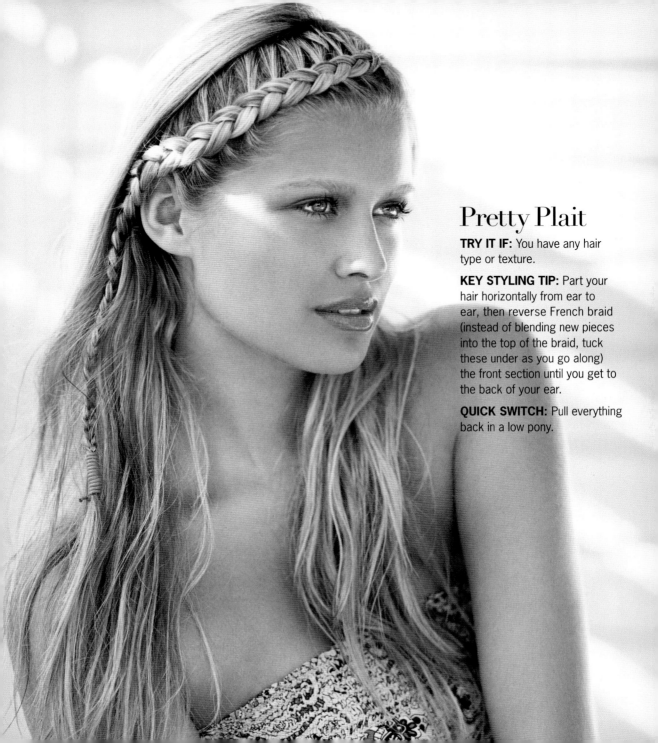

Pretty Plait

TRY IT IF: You have any hair type or texture.

KEY STYLING TIP: Part your hair horizontally from ear to ear, then reverse French braid (instead of blending new pieces into the top of the braid, tuck these under as you go along) the front section until you get to the back of your ear.

QUICK SWITCH: Pull everything back in a low pony.

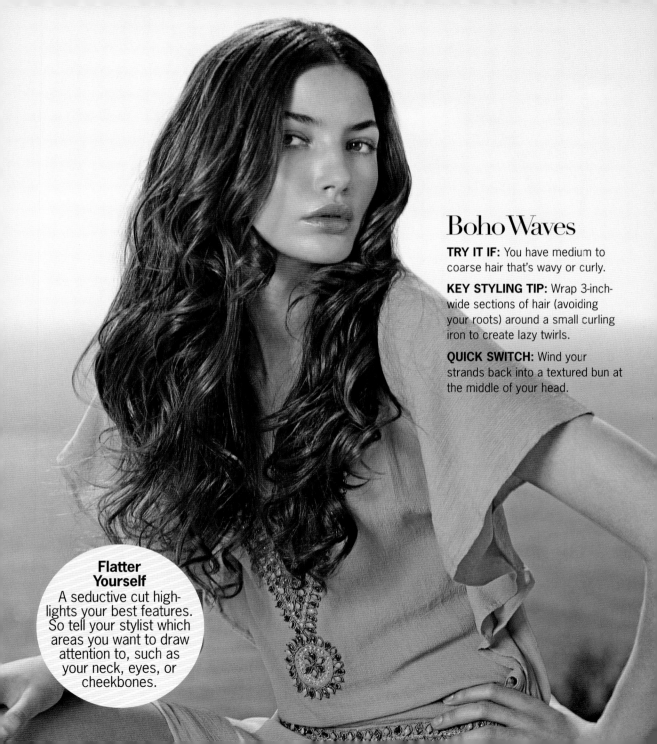

Boho Waves

TRY IT IF: You have medium to coarse hair that's wavy or curly.

KEY STYLING TIP: Wrap 3-inch-wide sections of hair (avoiding your roots) around a small curling iron to create lazy twirls.

QUICK SWITCH: Wind your strands back into a textured bun at the middle of your head.

Flatter Yourself
A seductive cut highlights your best features. So tell your stylist which areas you want to draw attention to, such as your neck, eyes, or cheekbones.

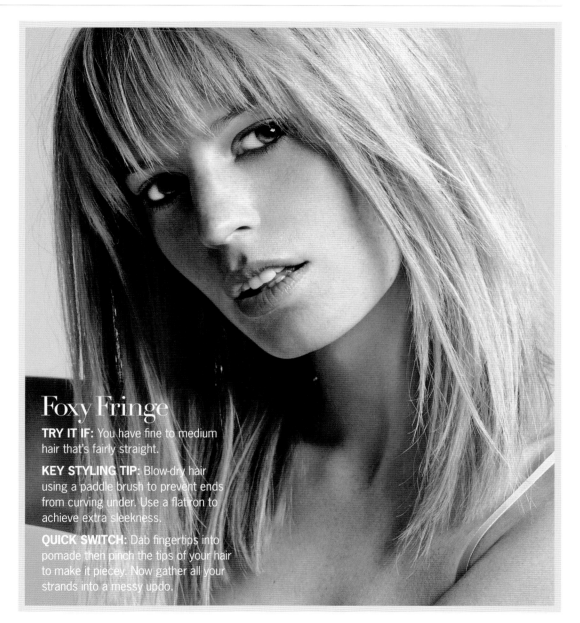

Foxy Fringe

TRY IT IF: You have fine to medium hair that's fairly straight.

KEY STYLING TIP: Blow-dry hair using a paddle brush to prevent ends from curving under. Use a flatiron to achieve extra sleekness.

QUICK SWITCH: Dab fingertips into pomade then pinch the tips of your hair to make it piecey. Now gather all your strands into a messy updo.

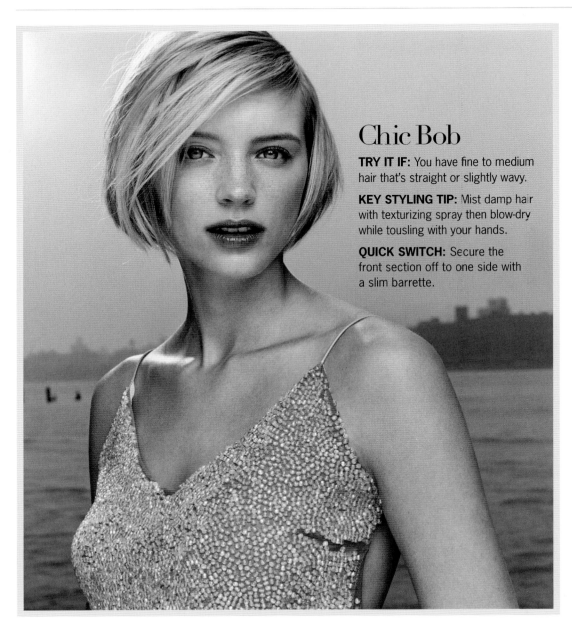

Chic Bob

TRY IT IF: You have fine to medium hair that's straight or slightly wavy.

KEY STYLING TIP: Mist damp hair with texturizing spray then blow-dry while tousling with your hands.

QUICK SWITCH: Secure the front section off to one side with a slim barrette.

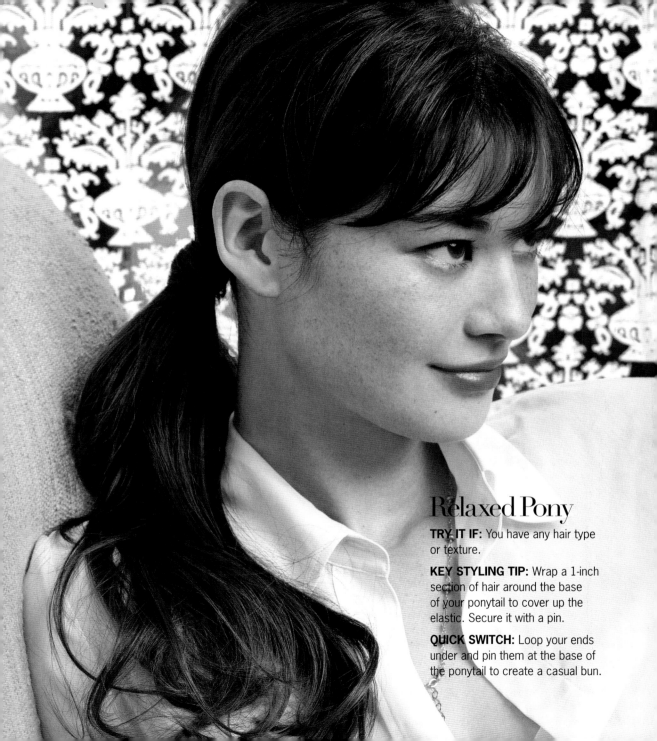

Relaxed Pony

TRY IT IF: You have any hair type or texture.

KEY STYLING TIP: Wrap a 1-inch section of hair around the base of your ponytail to cover up the elastic. Secure it with a pin.

QUICK SWITCH: Loop your ends under and pin them at the base of the ponytail to create a casual bun.

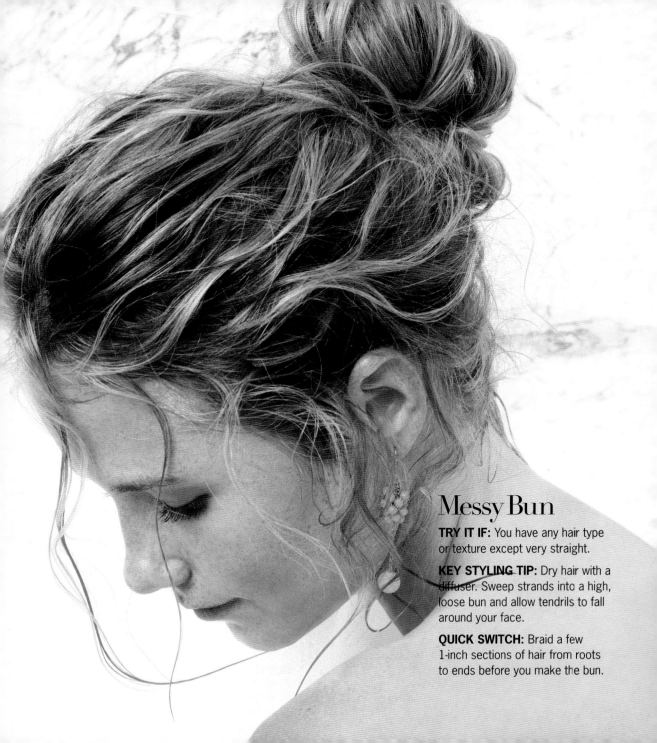

Messy Bun

TRY IT IF: You have any hair type or texture except very straight.

KEY STYLING TIP: Dry hair with a diffuser. Sweep strands into a high, loose bun and allow tendrils to fall around your face.

QUICK SWITCH: Braid a few 1-inch sections of hair from roots to ends before you make the bun.

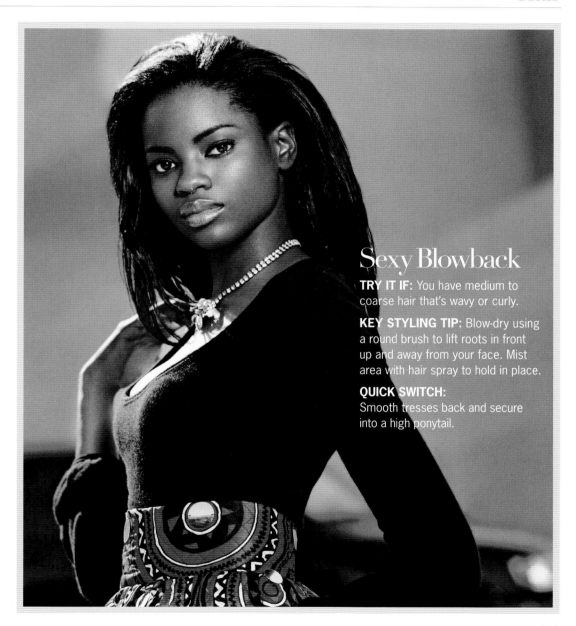

Sexy Blowback

TRY IT IF: You have medium to coarse hair that's wavy or curly.

KEY STYLING TIP: Blow-dry using a round brush to lift roots in front up and away from your face. Mist area with hair spray to hold in place.

QUICK SWITCH: Smooth tresses back and secure into a high ponytail.

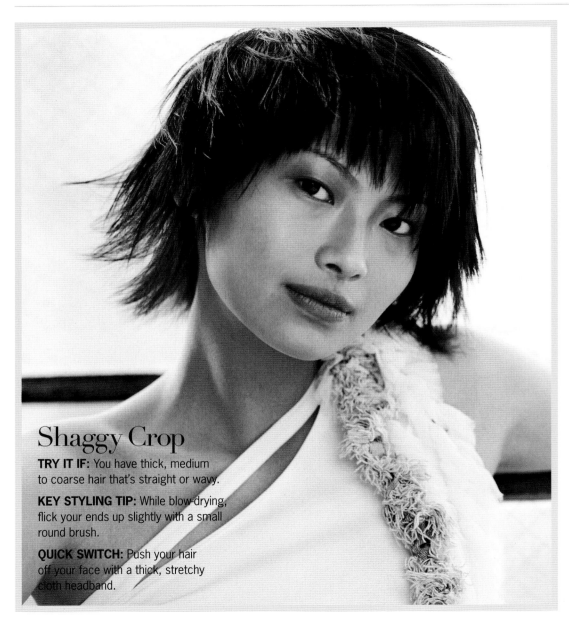

Shaggy Crop

TRY IT IF: You have thick, medium to coarse hair that's straight or wavy.

KEY STYLING TIP: While blow-drying, flick your ends up slightly with a small round brush.

QUICK SWITCH: Push your hair off your face with a thick, stretchy cloth headband.

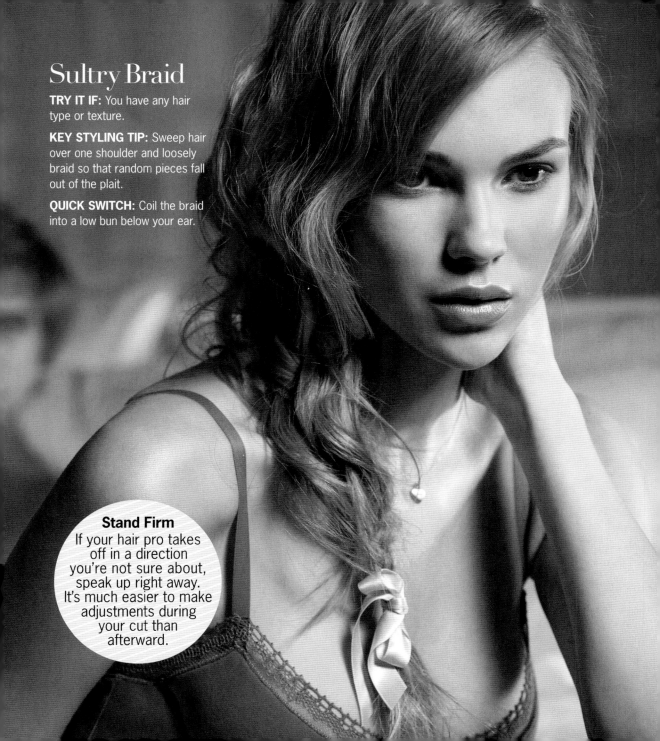

Sultry Braid

TRY IT IF: You have any hair type or texture.

KEY STYLING TIP: Sweep hair over one shoulder and loosely braid so that random pieces fall out of the plait.

QUICK SWITCH: Coil the braid into a low bun below your ear.

Stand Firm
If your hair pro takes off in a direction you're not sure about, speak up right away. It's much easier to make adjustments during your cut than afterward.

Body

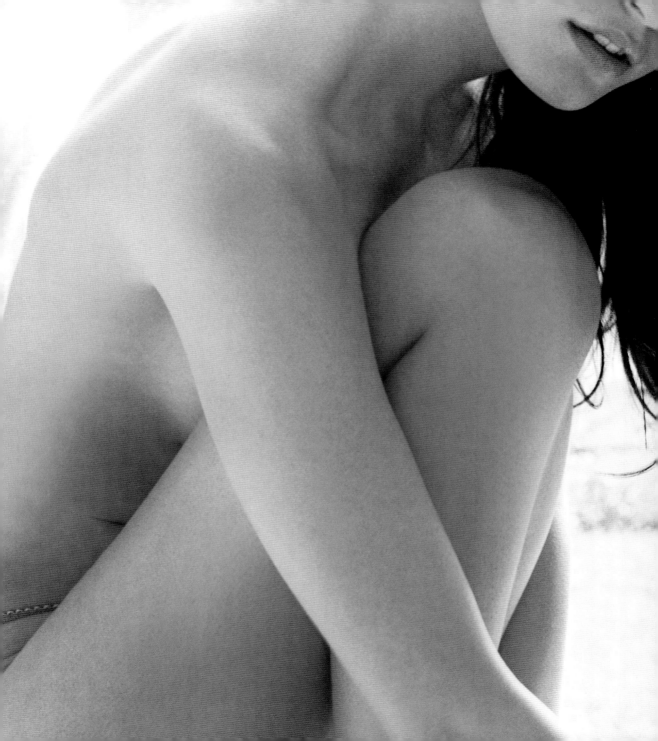

SECRETS OF

A Sexy Body

Your body is the biggest beauty canvas you have. So treat it right, girl! That means banishing breakouts (hey, buttne happens!), keeping your skin baby soft, and showing it off with sexy bronzers. And for those below-the-belt parts that are kept under wraps (well, most of the time), we'll give you tips on grooming your bikini line. So read on for the moves that'll make you glow literally from head to toe.

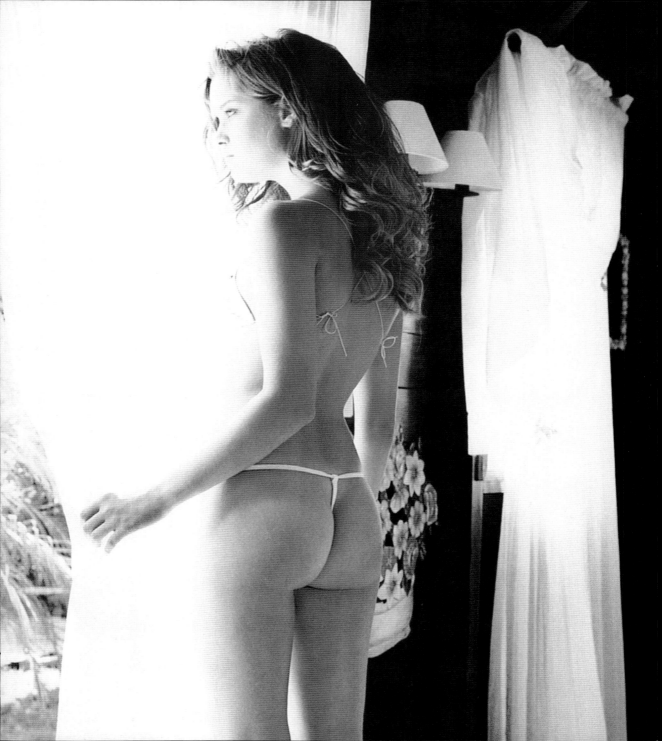

SOFTEN YOUR SKIN

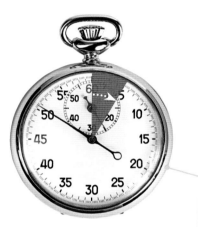

A beautiful body starts with silky-smooth skin. The tips you're about to read will get every inch of your flesh totally touchable.

■ Choose the Right Loot

There are about 3,000 products that promise to make your birthday suit supersoft, so we'll make this easy: Head straight for the body lotions with alpha hydroxy, glycolic, or lactic acids, which eat up dry, scaly skin cells. It's also a good idea to keep your showers on the short side (no longer than 10 minutes), use warm rather than hot water, and lather up with a hydrating body wash (look for one with glycerin or shea butter).

■ Lock in Moisture—Fast

The prime time to lube up: immediately following a shower. "Any longer than three to five minutes after you step out and the moisture will evaporate from your skin before your cream can seal it in," says dermatologist Elizabeth Tanzi, codirector of the Washington Institute of Dermatologic Laser Surgery, in Washington, D.C.

SEXY SECRET

Moisturizing Method

How you apply your body lotion is almost as important as when. Denise Vitello, director of the Mandarin Oriental hotel spa in New York City, uses a massagelike technique: She slowly moves her hands in circles toward the heart, which she says boosts blood flow for an allover flush.

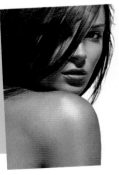

Buff to Get Buttery

Sloughing a few times a week is crucial to maintaining satiny skin, but you have to pick the right scrubber. Formulas with sugar are ideal for dry, sensitive skin since the granules are small, round, and dissolve quickly, says Gretchen Monahan, owner of G Spa and Grettacole day spa in Boston. Versions with salt are better for thicker, tougher skin (like your knees and elbows), since the granules are coarser and take longer to disintegrate in water.

So once you choose a type that's right for your bod, spa guru Cornelia Zicu says to spend about two minutes on each major body part, starting at the shoulders and ending at the toes, paying extra attention to your legs (they have the most real estate). "Rub a clean hand over each part until there are no flakes," she says.

BARE-IT-ALL BODY SECRETS

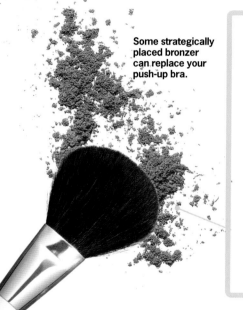

Some strategically placed bronzer can replace your push-up bra.

■ Beautify Your Bust

Those face masks you love so much can be beneficial to other body parts. "I use them on the neck and chest too," says Nicole Pozzetti, a paramedical aesthetician at TruSkin Clinical Spa, in NYC. "The skin there is delicate, and most masks contain gentle ingredients, such as clay and fruit extracts." For maximum benefits, Pozzetti says to rub the mask in using a technique called *effleurage* (French for "to touch lightly"), gliding your fingertips across your skin with swift, fluttery upward strokes. "This increases circulation and speeds up absorption," she explains.

Once your chest and décolletage are tended to, it's time to play up your most feminine assets (yes, we're talking about your breasts). With a large brush, dust bronzer in the hollow between your twins, then sweep a bit of pale shimmer over the tops of them. This creates visual depth and makes the round parts look fuller.

YOU SHOULD KNOW...
Supermarket Smoothers

Get this: Some budget ingredients can give you the same results as pricier potions. Add a handful of granulated sugar into a store-bought scrub to make it grittier. Or spike your body cream with a bit of honey to make it even more moisturizing. Another homespun tip: Squeeze half a lemon into the bath—the juice has natural acids that will brighten your skin.

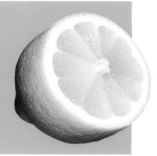

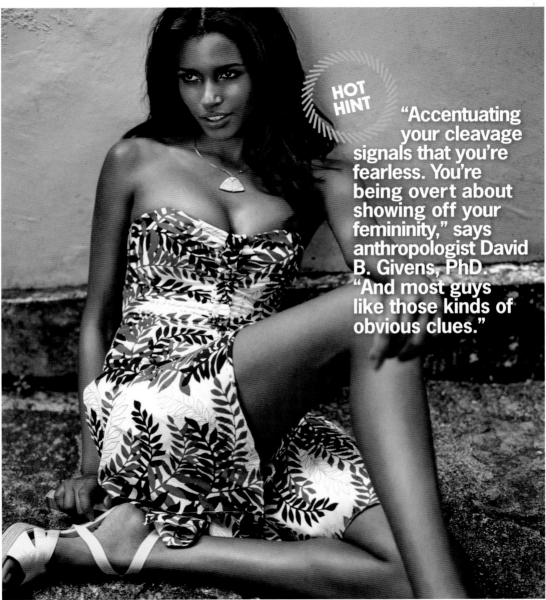

HOT HINT

"Accentuating your cleavage signals that you're fearless. You're being overt about showing off your femininity," says anthropologist David B. Givens, PhD. "And most guys like those kinds of obvious clues."

GET A PERFECT BIKINI LINE

A flawless bikini line is essential—but you hate the pain and upkeep, right? Here are some moves that'll make down-there grooming a breeze whether you decide to shave or wax.

If You Shave…

- Make sure your blade is sharp and clean. Razors that have at least three blades are best at not leaving a single hair behind.

- Try a transparent shaving gel. It allows you to see clearly where you're going. Too much foam can create a visibility issue.

- To reduce irritation, shave in the direction of hair growth at the end of your shower when the steam has softened your hair and skin.

- Prevent razor rash by applying a soothing witch-hazel toner postshaving. If you do get inflamed, use an antibiotic ointment.

A see-through gel will help you navigate your nether regions.

YOU SHOULD KNOW...

Eliminate Unsightly Bumps

Ingrown hairs are a bitch, but don't pick at them; just massage the area with a cotton ball soaked in a glycolic- or salicylic-acid face cleanser. "This sloughs off the skin's top layer and opens the follicle so the trapped hair can pass through," says New York City dermatologist Jeannette Graf, author of *Stop Aging, Start Living*.

If You Wax…

- If you're doing your own wax, the pros say to make sure your hair is at least one-quarter-inch long before you start.

- Looking for a completely sting-free at-home bikini waxing experience? Keep dreaming. But prepping your skin with a pat of cornstarch powder helps to at least dull the discomfort, says Gabrielle Ophals, co-owner of Haven spa in NYC. Cornstarch soaks up excess moisture that can make wax stick to skin (ouch!).

- When pulling off a wax strip, keep it as close and level to your skin as possible. In other words, don't pull upward.

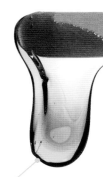

If waxing makes you wince, sprinkle on cornstarch powder first.

■ Sizzling Grooming Tip

Switching up your down-there style (returning to a full triangle if you've been bald or taking it all off if you're normally au natural) can give you a bedroom boost. Why? Changing looks signals to a guy that you'll also mix things up in bed, says sex educator Carol Queen, PhD.

49%

of guys love it when you're completely bare down there.

SOURCE: COSMO WEB POLL

SEXY SECRET

Down-There Dos

Give your guy a racy surprise by sculpting your bikini line into a saucy shape, like a lightning bolt or a heart. Buy a stenciling kit or use a bright lip liner to draw your shape, then shave around it.

127

SHAVE YOUR WAY TO SEXIER LEGS

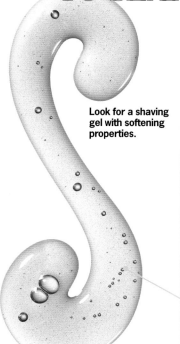

Look for a shaving gel with softening properties.

- For the kind of legs that have songs written about them, start by upgrading your razor. The best way to shave, says Cindy Barshop, founder of Completely Bare Spas in New York and Palm Beach, Florida, is with a three- or four-blade razor. "It cuts hairs in a single pass so you don't have to drag the blade over your skin repeatedly."

- Most of us grab the razor in the shower and get right to work. "But it's better to save shaving for last," says dermatologist Jeannette Graf. "The steam softens the hair, so removal is easier." For the best technique, experts say to hold skin taut and shave in the opposite direction of hair growth. When tackling sensitive areas, like the inner thighs, go with the grain to avoid ingrowns, advises Dr. Graf.

- Lather with the right stuff. Shaving creams with lubricating ingredients, such as silicone, oil, and cellulose gum, can help ward off annoying redness and irritation since they soften the hair and allow the razor to glide right over your skin, says Ni'Kita Wilson, a cosmetics chemist at Cosmetech Laboratories, in Fairfield, New Jersey. Scan product labels to find these smoothers.

SEXY SECRET
Smoother for Longer

If you have the patience and the pain threshold, try waxing your legs. "You're uprooting the hair from the follicle, as opposed to shaving it off at the surface, so you stay bare for a few weeks rather than a few days," says Bliss spa pro Ann Marie Cilmi.

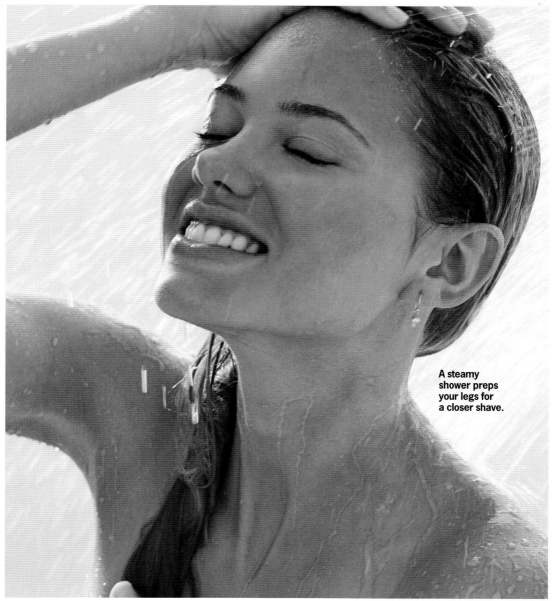

A steamy shower preps your legs for a closer shave.

HOW TO FAKE
A GREAT TAN

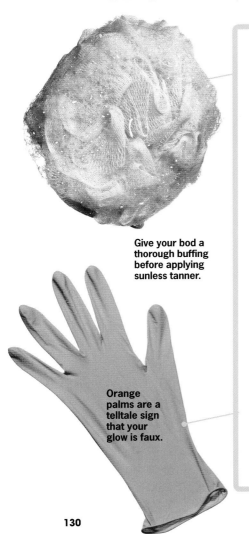

Give your bod a thorough buffing before applying sunless tanner.

Orange palms are a telltale sign that your glow is faux.

1. Scrub Your Skin

The golden rule of self-tanning is to exfoliate your entire body first. Skip this crucial step and you risk uneven, blotchy results. Pay extra attention to really dry spots like your elbows and knees.

2. Enhance Your Base

If your body is crypt-keeper pale, use a gradual self-tanner. "Ingredients in the cream react with the skin's amino acids to produce natural-looking brown pigments," says Dr. Graf. Your tone should peak in five to seven days. At that point, start applying the lotion every other day to maintain your gleam.

3. Get Instant Results

If you want a tanned look this second, your best bet is a bronzing oil that you can swipe on before going out. The effects only stick around until your next shower though. For something with more staying power, try a tinted mousse or a towelette with sunless tanner (which are less streaky than lotions and creams). Both stain your skin a golden hue, and the color lasts about a week.

4. Put on the Gloves

Before applying any tanner, pull on Latex (if you're not allergic) gloves. "That way, your palms won't soak up any color meant for your body," says spa owner Cindy Barshop. If you don't have gloves, wash your hands with soap when you're done. Put a dab of tanner on the top of each hand and rub them together so they're not completely pale.

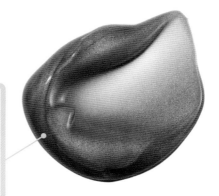

5. Use Broad Strokes

Make sure your body isn't greasy from any residual body cream, which can block the tanner from absorbing fully. Then spread the product on with uniform swipes in all directions. For knees and elbows, dilute the tanner with moisturizer. These dry spots absorb more color and can turn darker than the rest of your body. Also, skip spots where the sun don't shine, like your heels and soles, says Susie Hatton of Chocolate Sun tanning salon in Santa Monica, California.

6. Tone Down Any Streaks

If you end up with a few orange smudges, don't panic. A quick shower should fade them away. "If not, add a cup of milk to a bath," says Hatton. "The lactic acids help take down the color." If ankles, knees, or elbows are your only problem, buff away mess-ups with the fine side of a well-worn emery board or lighten them up with a bit of cream facial bleach left on for two to three minutes, says Dr. Graf.

Golden
***and* Toned**
Mix liquid bronzer
with a firming body
cream. The combo
will temporarily
tighten your skin and
make you glow.

SEXY SECRET

Gleamy, Dreamy Skin

For an instant shot of sexiness, swipe on a dry body oil after your faux tan has developed. You'll get a sexy, honey-hued shine. Be sure to let it seep in completely before getting dressed.

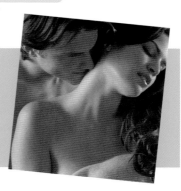

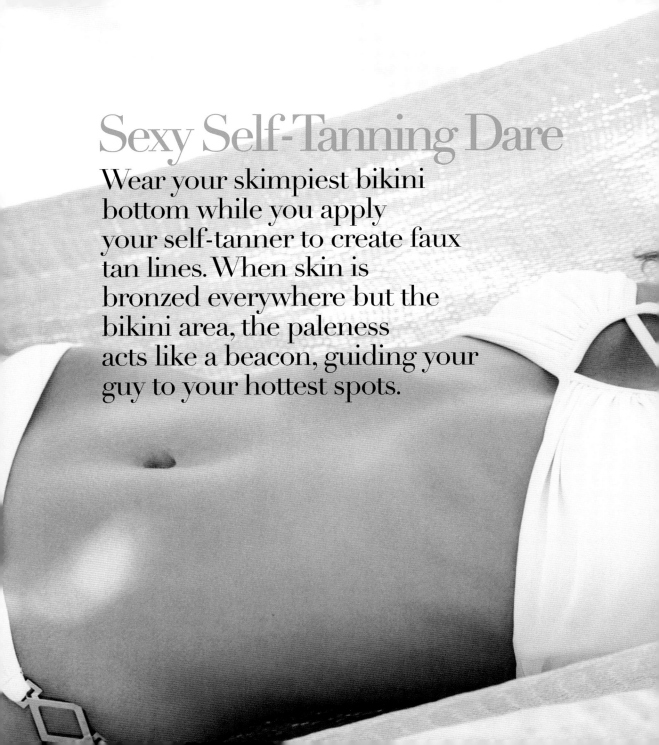

Sexy Self-Tanning Dare

Wear your skimpiest bikini bottom while you apply your self-tanner to create faux tan lines. When skin is bronzed everywhere but the bikini area, the paleness acts like a beacon, guiding your guy to your hottest spots.

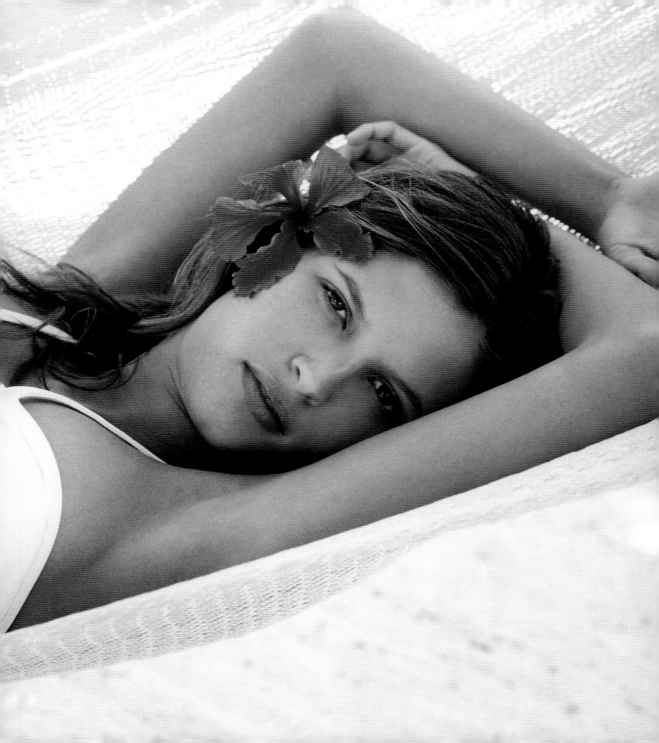

MAKE YOUR GAMS GLISTEN

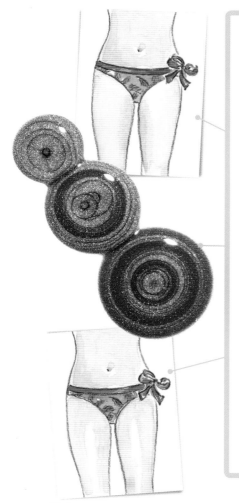

Even supermodels rely on some stealth beauty tricks to score longer, leaner looking legs (we swear!). Here, makeup artist Linda Hay reveals the backstage moves she has used on the Victoria's Secret girls before they hit the runway.

1 Contour With Self-Tanner

To create the appearance of muscle tone and definition, use a self-tanner that's a shade or two deeper than your natural color just on your inner thighs. This will also make your thighs look slightly smaller since just like dark clothes, dark skin can minimize your size.

2 Camouflage Imperfections

After self-tanning, give your legs an allover mist with an aerosol bronzer to blend away any obvious streaks and hide bruises or unsightly veins. If your feet are paler than your legs, hit the tops of them with the spray too so it doesn't look like you're wearing brown leggings.

3 Slim Your Stems

Dust a thin line of shimmer powder down the fronts and backs of your thighs and shins. Sprinkling it all over will only make legs look bigger than they actually are (*eek!*). Silver or pale pink glimmer looks prettiest on paler skin tones, whereas a champagne or gold version is most flattering on medium to dark skin tones.

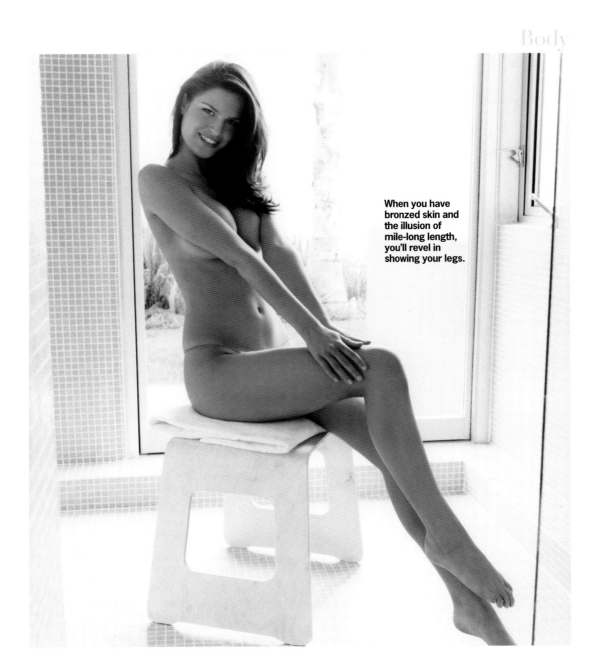

When you have bronzed skin and the illusion of mile-long length, you'll revel in showing your legs.

FIXES FOR BODY BUMMERS

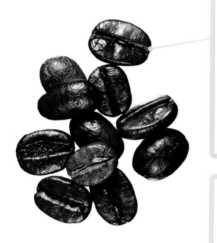

■ Outsmart Dimples

Unfortunately, there's no magic cure for cellulite, but most derms agree that lotions with caffeinated ingredients (like coffee, guarana, and tea) can boost circulation and reduce puckering temporarily. Another effective idea: Take a natural-bristle dry body brush and, starting at your ankles, rub upward, says Chantal Sanders, director of spa and boutique development for Clarins. This stimulates lymphatic drainage, which may ease puffiness. (It also helps to eat less salt.)

■ Banish Backne (and Buttne)

To ward off new spots while dealing with existing ones, use a body wash that has the pore-unclogging ingredient salicylic acid. Let the cleanser sit on your skin for a few minutes before rinsing to reap all the anti-acne benefits, says El Segundo, California, derm Howard Murad. Postshower, apply the same spot-treatment you use on your face (it should contain 2 percent salicylic acid, or sulfur).

SEXY SECRET

How to Hide a Hickey

Got a love bite on your neck? You naughty girl! To cover it up, use one of those greenish-yellow color-corrective concealers that counteract redness. Dab a bit over the most intense part of the spot, then apply a light layer of your regular foundation on top.

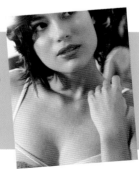

■ Prevent Boob Sweat

Curb ta-ta swelter before it starts by swiping a clear antiperspirant under your breasts prior to getting dressed, says celeb stylist June Ambrose. It's also a good idea to wear a cotton bra since it will absorb body moisture better than synthetic versions.

If you don't want "the girls" getting all hot and bothered, get a bra in a breathable fabric.

■ Keep Underarms Dry

Sweating isn't sexy (unless it's between the sheets). To make your antiperspirant more powerful, apply it before bedtime since it's absorbed better at night. Then glide on two more layers in the morning. You should stay dry all day.

■ Lose the Bruises

If you tag yourself on the corner of a table or a wall, ice the area first to prevent swelling. Then obscure the mark using a thick, creamy salmon or peach concealer, which neutralizes the bluish tint.

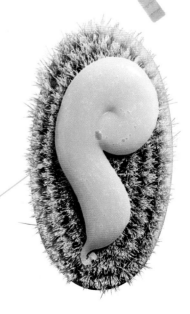

■ Ditch "Chicken Skin"

Those ugly red bumps on your arms are skin cells that build up around hair follicles. Slough them with a scrub that contains glycolic, lactic, or azelaic acids, says Kansas City derm Audrey Kunin.

TIPS FOR USING BODY BLING

How can you feel anything but pretty using a puff like this?

■ Taste as Sweet as You Look
Instead of using a regular shimmer body lotion or powder to play up your neckline and collarbone, go with a flavored formula. Your guy will get a yummy surprise when he goes in for a nuzzle.

TRY THIS TRICK!

Get the Right Amount of Sheen

Just like perfume and makeup, body shimmer should be used with restraint during daylight hours. To stay on the subtle side, mix up your own glimmer lotion. To do: Add a pinch of shimmer powder to your body lotion, says Nona Daron, owner of Flying Beauticians Day Spa in San Francisco. Smooth the combo on your legs only. On nights out, you can take it up a notch and double the dose of powder to about a teaspoon. Slather it on your arms, legs, and chest.

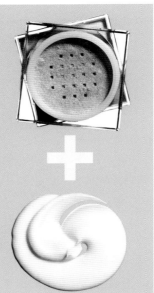

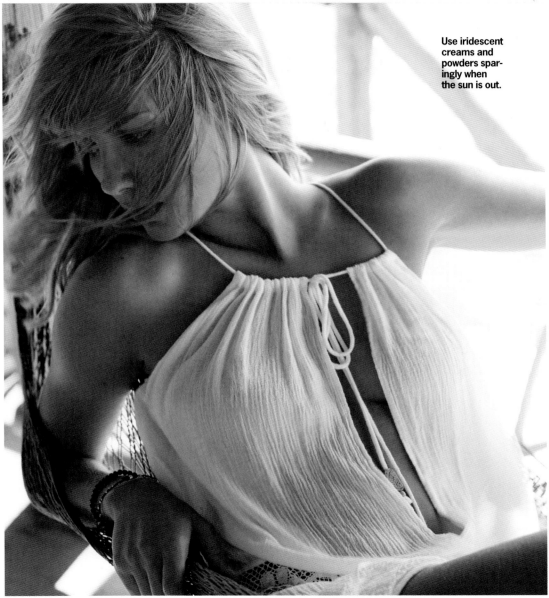

Use iridescent creams and powders sparingly when the sun is out.

Fragrance

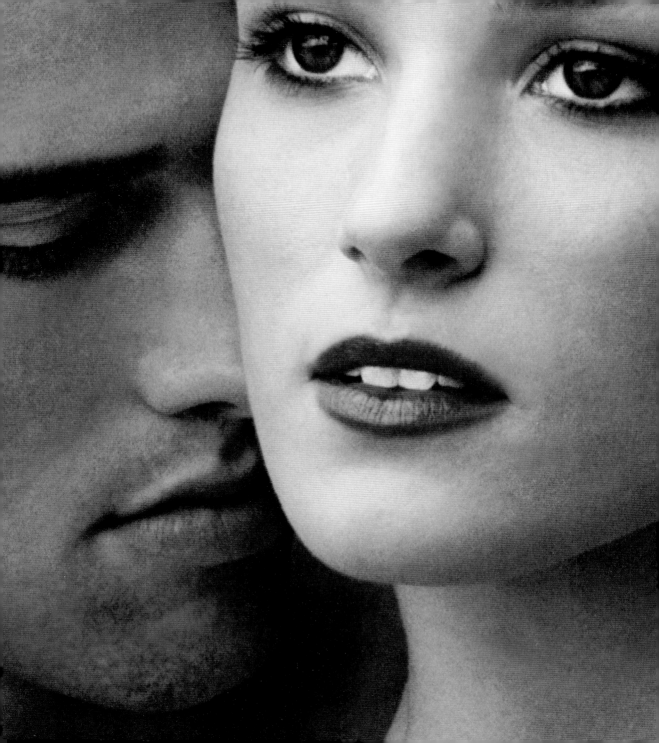

Seductive Scent

■ If you think fragrance is just the finishing touch on your primping routine, you're selling it way short. Scent has some impressive capabilities: According to scientific research, a few spritzes of a pretty potion can make you feel more alluring, put you in a sensual mood, and even affect a man's level of attraction to you. In fact, Cosmo has polled tons of guys to find out just how hot and bothered your fragrance can get them. Once you learn to harness the full potential of your perfume, it'll never be an afterthought again.

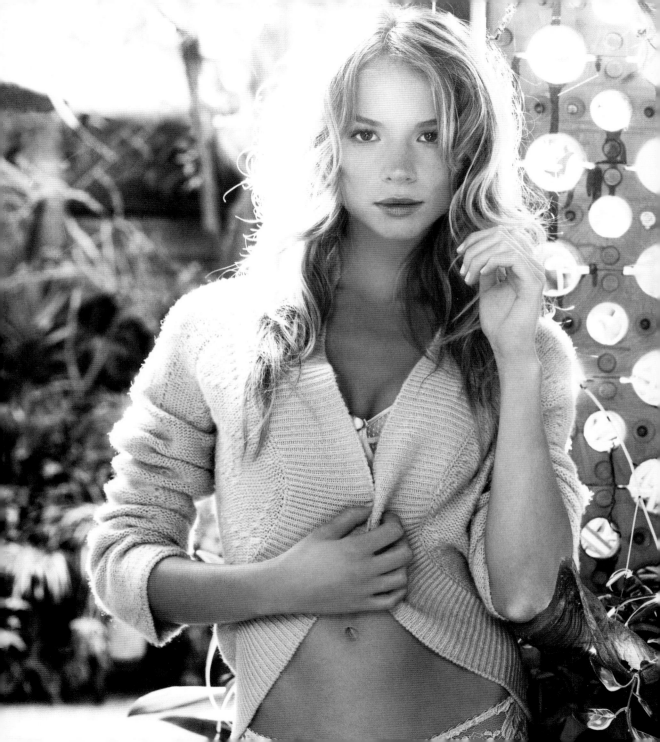

WHAT DIFFERENT AROMAS SAY—AND DO

FLORALS. Flowers like rose, lily, tuberose, and gardenia have historically been associated with love and femininity, says Alan Hirsch, MD, director of Chicago's Smell and Taste Treatment and Research Foundation. That means even men find a floral scent romantic.

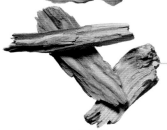

ORIENTALS AND MUSKS. Intense notes—such as sandalwood, amber, and musk—stand out because they're exotic, says Craig Warren, PhD, scientific affairs director of the Sense of Smell Institute in NYC. As a result, guys associate these scents with mystery.

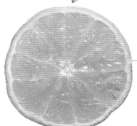

CITRUS AND FRUITS. Fruity fragrances can boost your mood since they're lively and energizing, says Warren. Also, juicy aromas like berry, apple, orange, and peach send out happy, positive vibes, which is always an attractive quality to guys.

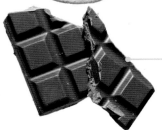

GOURMANDS. Tasty scents like chocolate, vanilla, and crème brûlée are comforting and familiar, so they connect to a man's emotional cravings, says Dr. Hirsch. All the more reason why he'll want to nibble on you.

■ Finding the Right Fragrance

Choosing a scent is like picking out the perfect piece of lingerie—it's a tricky decision because what you go with can say a lot about your personality. Here, some helpful hints to make the hunt easier.

Shop in the morning. Your nose is less tired from sniffing all day and isn't saturated with other smells, says Pascal Gaurin, senior perfumer at International Flavors and Fragrances.

Don't eat spicy foods the night before browsing. They can make a scent smell more intense than it should on your skin, according to Rochelle Bloom, president of the Fragrance Foundation.

Know your audience. Does your beau like spicy or citrus scents? Bring him with you so you don't have to guess what will turn him on.

Ask the salesperson for a free sample of a perfume and wear it for a few days to see if you really love it.

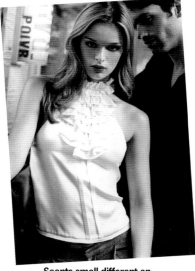

Scents smell different on everyone, so only buy a fragrance that you've tested on yourself.

SEXY SECRET

Good Enough to Eat

According to a Cosmo poll, **36 percent** of guys love a dessertlike scent on a first date. Runner-up scents: 27 percent preferred fruity notes, while 18 percent found florals appealing.

Smart Spritzing
Women were rated higher in intelligence and friendliness when they wore perfume on a job interview.

SOURCE: *JOURNAL OF APPLIED PSYCHOLOGY*

145

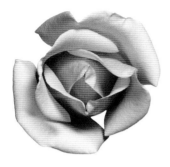

THE SCENT TO SPRITZ ON TONIGHT

Betcha didn't know that fragrance can intensify your mood. Before heading out for the night, tap into your vibe by answering the questions below. Then spray accordingly.

The outfit you are dying to pull on:
- ⓐ A slinky minidress and wedge heels
- ⓑ Jeans, a low-cut tee, and cute flats
- ⓒ A ruffled skirt, a camisole, and pumps

The makeup look you're planning to rock is:
- ⓐ Smoky eyes and pale lips.
- ⓑ Sun-kissed bronzer and clear lip gloss.
- ⓒ Shimmery eye shadow, rosy blush, and peach lipstick.

The playlist you queue up before going out:
- ⓐ Hits from obscure indie bands
- ⓑ Booty shakers from your fave R&B artists
- ⓒ Nostalgic pop classics

A few hours into the night, you can imagine yourself:
- ⓐ Locking eyes with a hot guy across the room.
- ⓑ Moving on from your first party and heading to the next.
- ⓒ Meeting up with your man for a late-night cocktail.

Your go-to drink for the night will probably be:
- ⓐ Whatever the bartender surprises you with.
- ⓑ Vodka with a splash of Red Bull.
- ⓒ Champagne or a fruity libation.

The ideal end to your evening is:
- ⓐ Trading texts with a hottie you met.
- ⓑ Watching the sun rise.
- ⓒ Crawling into bed with your man.

If You Answered...

 Mostly A's — Mysterious

The right fragrance: a musky oriental with sweet or spicy undertones that's as sensuous and unpredictable as you are

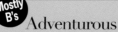 **Mostly B's** — Adventurous

The right fragrance: a bold citrus that boosts your energy but won't overpower your already upbeat mood

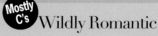 **Mostly C's** — Wildly Romantic

The right fragrance: a floral that's dreamy and inviting with a classic rose base and fruity modern top note

Not All Potions Are Created Equal

Fragrances come in many forms.
Here's the lowdown on each.

Eau de parfum. Because they contain a high concentration of perfume oil, eau de parfums are very intense.

Solid perfume. These balmlike formulas have a viscous texture, so they actually stick to the skin, which makes them last.

Eau de toilette. If you want a scent to be subtle, go with an eau de toilette—they have a low concentration of perfume oil.

Roller-ball perfume. Roller-ball fragrances are applied directly to the body, which allows them to be absorbed and released quickly.

Body cream. Layer a scented cream with a similar-smelling perfume to maximize it's barely-there payoff.

Scented hair mists. Hair mists have the potency of a fragrance, but they're specially formulated not to damage your mane.

Body spray. Body sprays leave a thin layer of fragrance on the skin, so they're a great way to freshen up postworkout.

Body powder. It's one of the softest, lightest forms of scent. Rub it onto your arms and legs after toweling off from the shower.

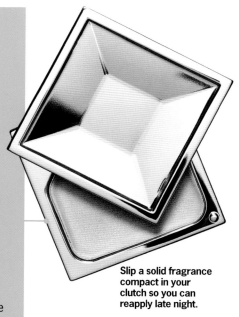

Slip a solid fragrance compact in your clutch so you can reapply late night.

Your nose is able to identify up to an amazing

10,000

different smells.

SOURCE: SCENT EXPERT
ALAN HIRSCH, MD

147

THE LINK BETWEEN SCENT AND SEDUCTION

Cosmo polled hundreds of hot-blooded men to find out what your fragrance can do to their senses. Sneak peek of the findings: It has a major impact!

84%
believe perfume has the power to turn them on or off.

Perfume arouses men on a very primal level, says Dr. Alan Hirsch. "Pleasant aromas can actually stimulate parts of the brain directly connected to sexual desire," he explains. And that can lead to some very lusty thoughts.

81%
think a woman's scent could boost her overall attractiveness.

He's already transfixed by your looks, but wearing a scent shows you're doing something extra special—and sensual—for him. "In that way, fragrance can enhance feelings and emotions," says Dr. Hirsch. It can even change our perceptions in the early days of dating.

42%
say they have fantasized about a woman's perfume.

While planting your panties in his bed will excite him, leaving a delicate trail of scent behind can drive him insane with desire. For even more impact, keep him guessing: For example, if you normally wear something floral, spritz a spicier blend on your sheets or lingerie.

35%
would sleep with a woman because her scent was appealing.

Since caveman days, the brain has been hardwired to size up potential mates simply based on scent, says Jeannette Haviland-Jones, PhD, professor of psychology at Rutgers University, in New Jersey. The body emits odors that spur us to hook up with fertile partners.

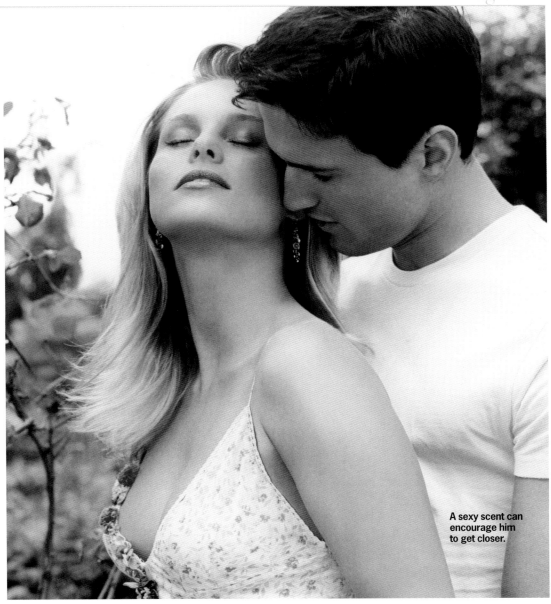

A sexy scent can encourage him to get closer.

How His Cologne Can Rev Your Engine

Sure, you can drive him crazy with your perfume, but what about the impact his scent has on you? "Smell is one of the first things you notice about a guy, and it can have a strong effect on your feelings for him," says New Jersey sensory psychologist Avery Gilbert. In fact, one study found that men's cologne, especially light, subtle versions, can enhance sexual physical arousal in women. Unlike heavy aromas, fresh men's scents may be best because they have "clean" notes women associate with getting intimate with a guy.

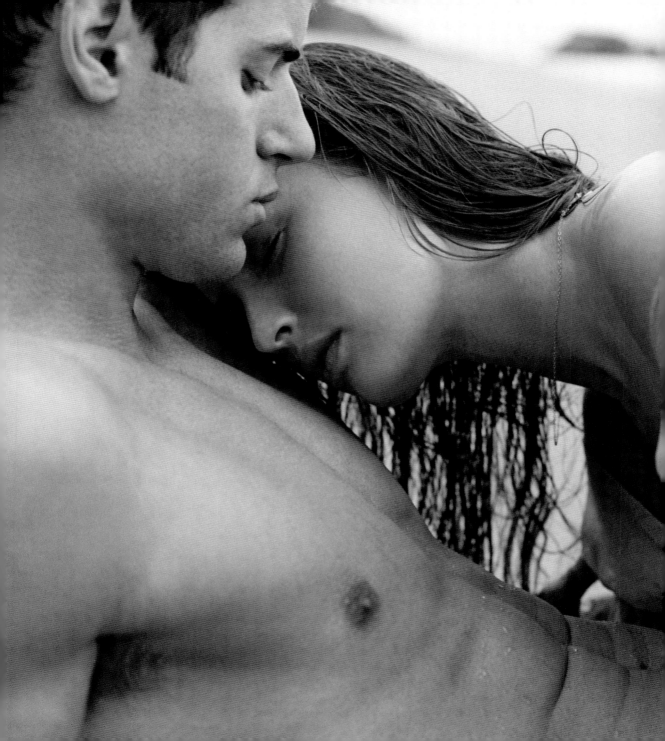

TRICKS TO FLAUNT
A FABULOUS SCENT

Pulse points to spritz:
- Behind your ears
- The inside of your wrists
- The nape of your neck
- Your belly
- Between your breasts
- The backs of your knees

■ Where to Wear It

We've all been told to dab perfume on our wrists for good reason: "Your pulse points are always a bit warmer than other areas of your body because the skin there is very thin and your blood runs very close to it," says Rachel Herz, PhD, author of *The Scent of Desire*. When fragrance hits these specific areas of your skin, the aromas are diffused into the air more powerfully." FYI: Your torso is a natural heat center too, so it's also a good area to hit with fragrance.

■ Avoid a Fragrance OD

The olfactory receptors in the brain become immune to most smells after about 15 minutes, warns Dr. Hirsch. That means you can't always trust your own nose to tell you when you're oversaturated...but it's obvious to others. To make sure you're not setting off scent alarms, apply the same amount—one to two dabs or mist the air and walk through the cloud—in the morning and before going out at night.

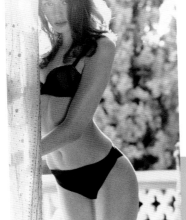

SEXY SECRET
Forespray Your Lingerie
Mist your bra and undies (except the crotch) with a sexy scent to give your guy an unexpected surprise when he goes to peel them off.

Smell Amazing All Day

Just like New Year's resolutions, perfumes have a way of fading fast. Tricks to make them last:

1 Pulse points give off the most heat to release fragrance, so definitely spray your scent on more than one of these sweet spots.

2 Dry skin can't hold scents well, so rub on a perfumed lotion first to hydrate and smell pretty.

3 Spritz a scent onto the inner lining of your clothes for a subtle whiff every time you move.

CUSTOMIZE YOUR BREW

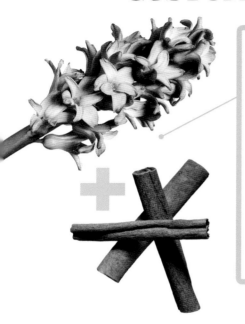

Invent your own fragrance by layering a few scents. We asked Debbie Wild, director of brand education and development for Jo Malone, for advice on creating a signature aroma. A few guidelines:

- Florals and spices combine to produce a sensual, alluring effect.

- Fragrances from the same family—a light floral with a basic floral, for example—give each other depth without changing the fundamental nature of either.

- A woody scent will give just the right boost to a citrus scent.

HOT TIP **When you're layering, spray on one fragrance, let your skin dry, then spray a different one on the same spot.**

Fun, Fearless Fragrance!

A martini isn't the only thing that makes a woman feel bolder. In a study, **97 percent** of women said wearing fragrance boosts their confidence in social situations. Research also shows that when women wear any pleasant fragrance (the exact scent doesn't matter), they project a more positive attitude, says Theresa Molnar, executive director of the Sense of Smell Institute.

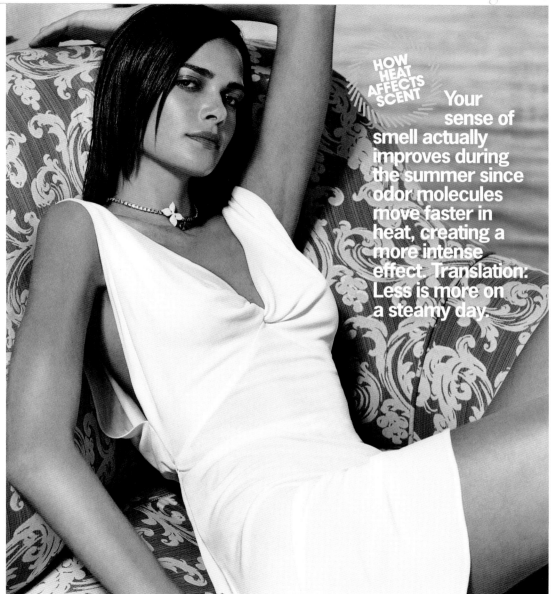

HOW HEAT AFFECTS SCENT Your sense of smell actually improves during the summer since odor molecules move faster in heat, creating a more intense effect. Translation: Less is more on a steamy day.

Nails

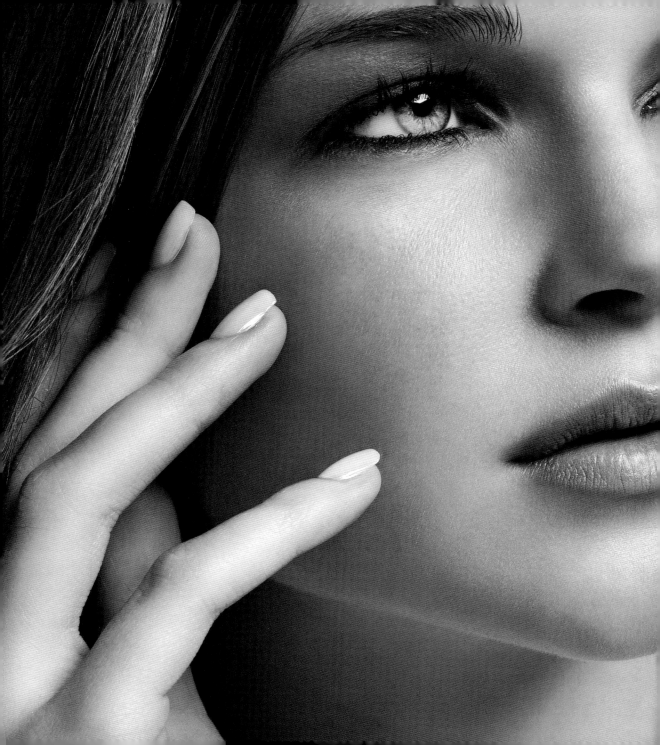

Perfect Nails

■ Nails may not be a guy's number one pick for a woman's sexiest feature, but trust us—they notice them. Whether you're using them to tickle him somewhere naughty or adorning them with a vixen-ish shade of polish, your talons can be a secret seduction weapon. And that's not all. Keeping your nails (on your fingers and toes) groomed and glossy can make you seem more sophisticated. Plus, a mani or pedi is a great way to pamper yourself. So buff up on these tips to make your hands and feet look their foxiest.

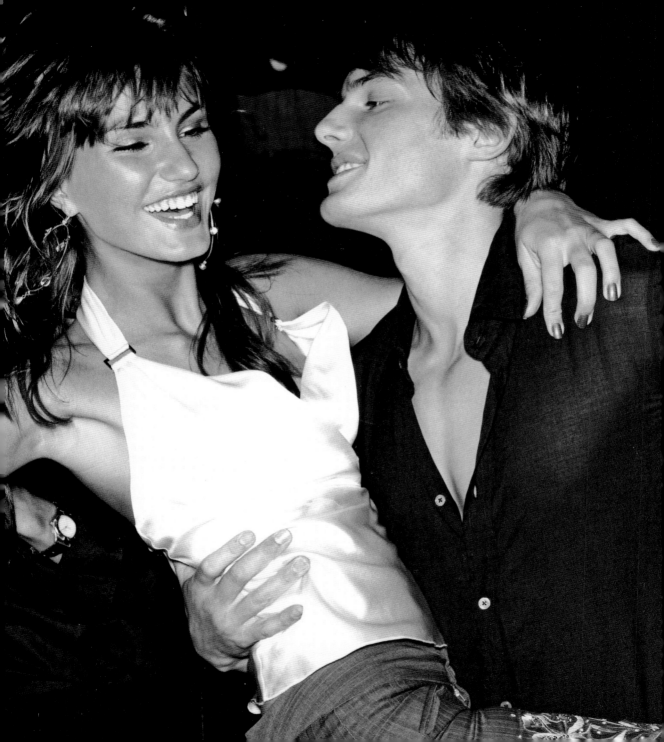

GET PRETTY HANDS

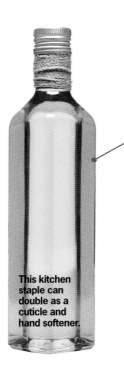

This kitchen staple can double as a cuticle and hand softener.

■ Pamper at Night

Your hands take a daily beating, but with some regular TLC you can keep them supple. Here's how: Before bed whip up a sugar scrub by combining two tablespoons of olive oil with two tablespoons of sugar, says Patricia Yankee Williams, nail technician for Dashing Diva salons. Massage it into your hands until the sugar begins to dissolve. Rinse off with warm water. Next, add a few drops of olive oil to a super-rich hand cream and rub it into your hands and cuticles. Slip on cotton gloves and wear them overnight. It's not the sexiest p.m. attire, but your hands will feel amazing in the morning.

■ Give Yourself a Hand

Relieve stress with this pressure-point rubdown. Use one of your thumbs to press the area between your other thumb and forefinger while breathing deeply for two minutes, says Ann Emich-Patton, senior consultant for Blu Spas in Scottsdale, Arizona. Then switch hands.

YOU SHOULD KNOW...

Quick Fix

It's easy to mend a broken nail as long as it isn't hanging by a thread, says Ji Baek, owner of Rescue Beauty Lounge, in NYC. Her talon-saving tip: Apply a dot of nail glue on top of the split, then cover with a tiny piece of tissue and seal it to your nail with another drop of glue. Let dry, then buff to a smooth finish.

PRO MANICURE TECHNIQUES

- In addition to cleaning nails with a non-oil-based polish remover before applying lacquer, the experts at Dashing Diva in NYC use a plush buffer to smooth out any ridges and refine the nail's surface.

- Slash your polish's drying time by slicking on two very thin coats, says celeb manicurist Deborah Lippmann. For the lightest application, wipe the brush against the neck of the bottle.

- To figure out if nails are one hundred percent dry, Jessica Vartoughian, founder of Jessica Cosmetics in Beverly Hills, says to apply cold water to one nail. If it glides off, you're good to go.

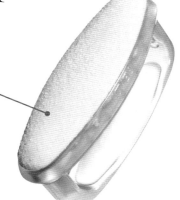

Gently buff your nails before painting them to make a manicure last longer.

Your Best Nail Shape

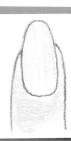

SQUARE
This look is best on medium-length nails.
TECHNIQUE
Drag the file straight across the top of the nail. Once that part is straight, you can curve the corners a bit by gently moving the fine side of the file vertically over the edges.

OVAL
This shape keeps short nails from looking stubby.
TECHNIQUE
Working in a clockwise motion, rub a file under your nail in an arch following the curve of your finger. Use the softer grain to file the edges into a crescent-moon shape.

TAPERED
This shape looks great if you have slim fingers and long nails.
TECHNIQUE
First, file your nails into soft ovals. Then, starting at the top of the nail, move the file straight down one side until you hit your finger. Repeat on the other side.

THE SEXIEST
LACQUER SHADE

When In Doubt, Go Red

There are a ton of polish colors out there, and many of them have their place in your beauty loot collection (e.g., pale pink for a job interview). But when it comes to looking sexy, traffic lights and sirens are red for a reason: It's the color that makes us stop in our tracks. Red and deep berry tones are the most sexually arousing, and they also convey courage. "Red is hot," says Lionel Tiger, PhD, professor of anthropology at Rutgers University. "It just is."

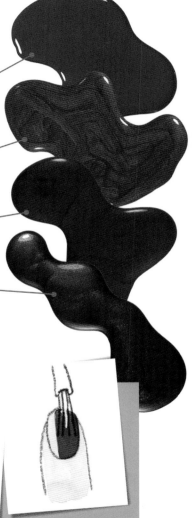

■ The Perfect Red for Your Skin Color

If your skin is light with yellow undertones,
opt for a warm coral or tomato red.

If your skin is light with blue undertones,
go for a cool rose red or deep berry red.

If your skin is medium,
a reddish violet hue provides a nice
contrast with olive complexions.

If your skin color is dark,
all reds look hot with African-American skin,
but a metallic formula will really pop.

How to Pull Off a Flawless Paint Job

Though it's hard to master a scarlet mani, it's so worth the effort. To do it right:

STEP 1. Start at the center of the nail, says Suzi Weiss-Fischmann, artistic director of OPI. This way, any excess paint will slide onto your nail, not your cuticles.

STEP 2. Apply a stroke of polish on either side of the first one, from the base to the tip. Wait two minutes, then apply a second coat following the same moves.

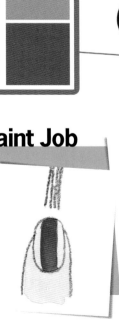

POLISH POINTERS

■ Pale Hue Hint
Prevent your light polish colors from yellowing in the sun with a UV-protectant topcoat. If it's too late, just buff away the top layer of your polish with a fine-grained file then apply a coat of clear lacquer.

■ Go Nude, Not Naked
A flesh-tone polish is the most practical hue—chips are undetectable, it goes with everything, and because it almost matches your skin, it'll elongate the look of your fingers, says nail pro Deborah Lippmann.

Use a neutral color when you're in a rush—any goofs will be harder to see.

■ Dress Up Your Mani
Slick a clear sparkly lacquer over your regular polish. It'll catch the light (and someone's eye) during a night out on the town.

SEXY SECRET

Fresh Twists on the French Manicure
A French manicure may be a classic look, but let's be honest—it's a bit old school for a pretty young thing like you. So swap the standard beige-and-matte-white combo for a softer baby pink polish as the base and a sheer shimmery white polish at the tip (keep the strip on the thin side), says New Jersey manicurist Skyy Hadley.

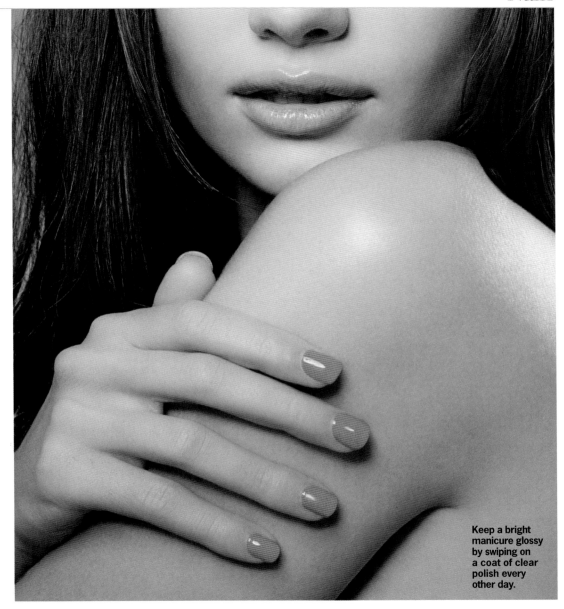

Keep a bright manicure glossy by swiping on a coat of clear polish every other day.

SOLE-SMOOTHING MOVES

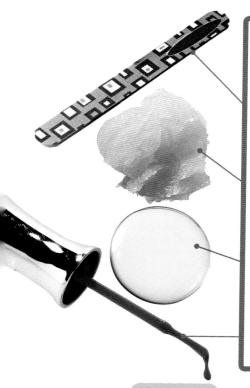

The Ultimate DIY Pedi

Pull off a pro job when you can't make it to the salon.

■ **Trim and File**
Cut toenails straight across and file away sharp corners, being careful not to round the edges, which can cause the nail to grow into the surrounding skin, warns dermatologist Jeannette Graf.

■ **Prime the Skin**
Gently buff away any calluses and rough spots with a pumice stone, then apply a smoothing foot scrub, suggests Julie Serquinia, owner of Paint Shop Beverly Hills nail salon.

■ **Soak It Up**
Push back your cuticles with a damp washcloth and rub in moisturizer and cuticle oil, letting them sink in for a minute or two. Wipe off any greasy residue that is left behind.

■ **Paint It On**
Apply a base coat, two layers of polish, and then a high-shine topcoat.

SEXY SECRET

A Special At-Home Treat

Soak your tootsies in a bowl of warm orange juice for 10 minutes (the acids are exfoliating), says Donna Perillo, owner of Sweet Lily Natural Nail Spa and Boutique, in NYC. Then rub your heels and other rough spots with a coarse foot scrub. Rinse it off and wrap hot towels over each foot for 5 minutes. Afterward, apply a thick cream.

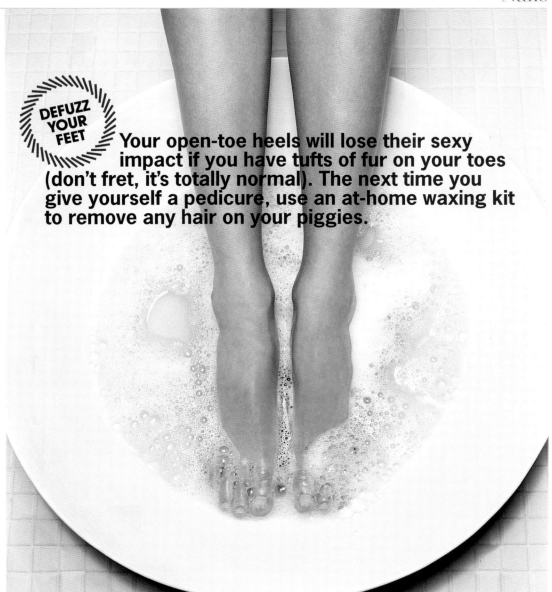

DEFUZZ YOUR FEET Your open-toe heels will lose their sexy impact if you have tufts of fur on your toes (don't fret, it's totally normal). The next time you give yourself a pedicure, use an at-home waxing kit to remove any hair on your piggies.

SEXY TOES ALL YEAR LONG

Just as your wardrobe changes with the seasons, so should your pedicure. Here, Essie Weingarten, creator of Essie Cosmetics, tells you which hue looks hottest, depending on the time of year.

Summer
Vibrant shades of coral pop against all skin tones.

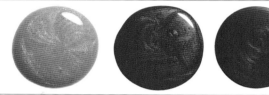

Fall
Rich brownish reds compliment darker fall clothing.

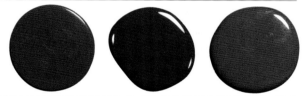

Winter
Dramatic shades of red and purple match the mood of winter and look hot with a little black dress.

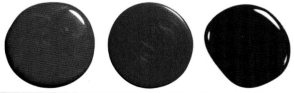

Spring
Bright pinks and berry colors go well with spring's flirty vibe.

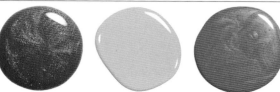

Daily Care

When you know that your feet are going to be front and center—like on vacay, during sandal season, or when you're playing footsie in bed—you should pay extra attention to them.

Slough your soles every night with a foot-specific scrub (they're grittier than regular body versions) or use a callus smoother, advises nail expert Jan Arnold, cofounder of CND hand and feet products. Then apply an alpha-hydroxy acid–infused foot lotion for simultaneous exfoliating and softening action. When you have a guy-free night, slather on an extra-thick layer of the lotion and pad around in slippers for a few hours or wear a pair of cotton socks overnight. You'll wake up to baby-bottom-soft tootsies.

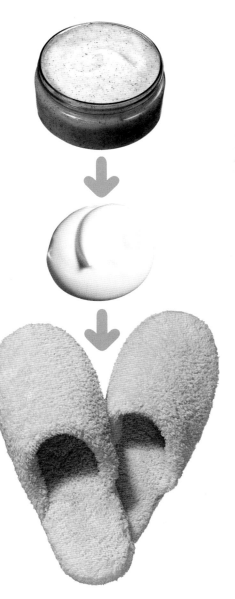

Pampering

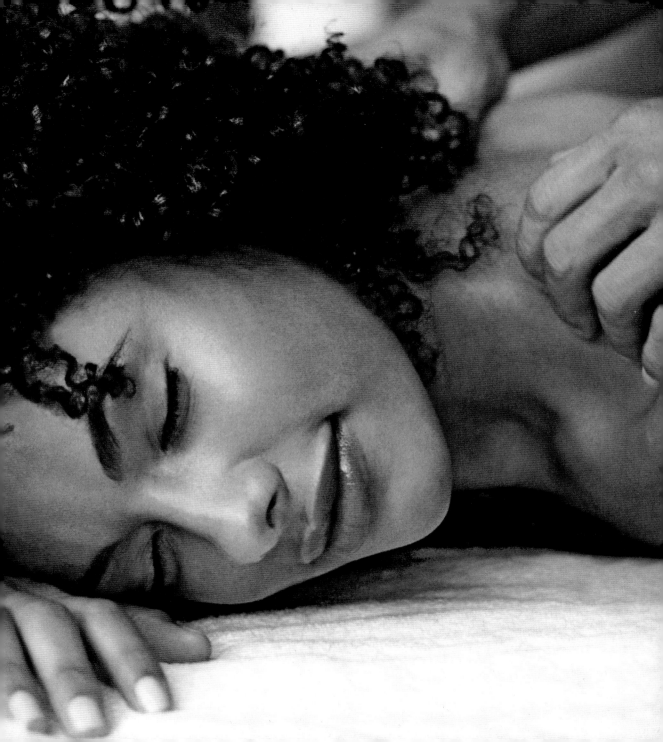

Spoiling Yourself Spa-Style

■ Whether you have been to a spa or only dream of going to one, you can imagine how blissful you'd feel and how beautiful you'd look if you could regularly indulge in the treatments those kinds of retreats supply. Spas use special tricks and ingredients to relax your body (and mind!) and make your skin glow. What's surprising is that you can actually achieve similar results at home…if you know the spa secrets we're about to divulge here.

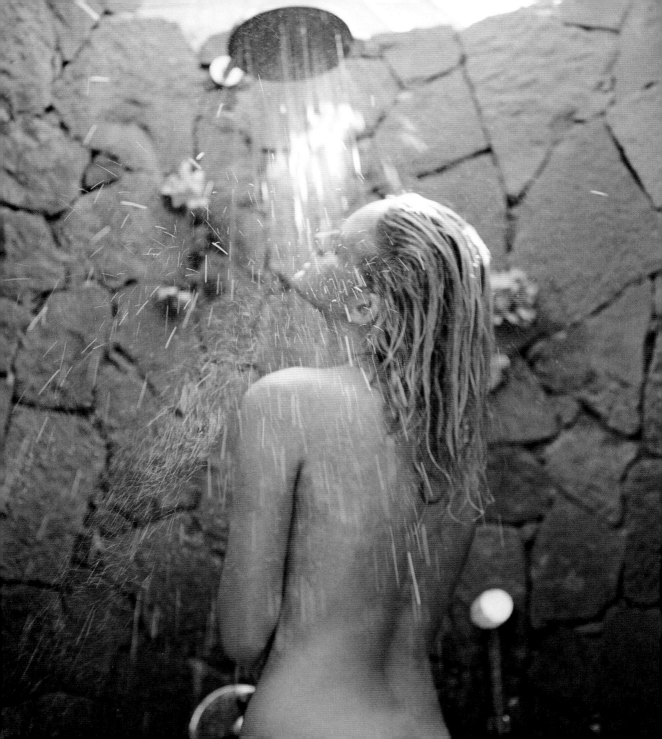

SOOTHING SHOWERS

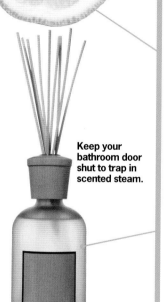

Keep your bathroom door shut to trap in scented steam.

A get-clean-quick rinse is fine during the week. But when you have the time to spare, try one of these totally divine, skin-silkening rituals.

Soften up with lemon. Squeeze fresh lemon juice on a wet washcloth and rub it against your skin, advises Kimberly Gambill, spa director at the Parker Palm Springs Estate, in California. The citric acid buffs while the rind oil moisturizes.

Toy with temperature. Top off a shower by turning the water on cold for 30 seconds to really get your circulation going, says Jason Harler, spa director of the Standard hotel in Miami Beach, where clients are encouraged to hop between hot deluge showers and cool-plunge pools.

Create a sensual aroma. Place a satchel of potpourri behind your showerhead. As the mist rises, the scent will fill up the area. Or put a fragrance diffuser (like the one shown here) in your bathroom.

Give yourself a tingling head rub. Most spas max out their services by combining treatments. So add a scalp-stimulating massage to your body-buffing shower. Apply a cooling peppermint essential oil to your roots, then rub firmly with your fingertips. For added bliss, knead your temples and earlobes.

SEXY SECRET

Just Add Oil
You've been lathering up with soap and soaking in bubbles since you were a baby, but if you mix in a sexy, scented essential oil, you get a shower or bath that's especially luxe.

BLISSFUL BATHS

These decadent tub strategies can turn an ordinary soak into an enchanting, tension-relieving, spalike experience.

- **Submerge your ears.** It's an ideal way to destress and chill out, says Shannon Curry of the Miraval Life in Balance resort, in Arizona. "You can hear your heartbeat and your breathing, which lends a calming meditative quality," she says. Keep your ears under for just a few minutes at a time.

- **Save your soles (or his) with a watsu stroke.** Watsu, a form of muscle-relaxing shiatsu massage that is performed underwater, is a huge spa hit. "At home, try it out on your feet. You'll see that the warm water makes a foot rub even more amazing," says Aida Thibiant, owner of the Thibiant Beverly Hills Day Spa. Use your thumb to press small circles from the base of your toes to your heels.

- **Follow a 20-minute soak with a quick shower.** Because dead surface-skin cells have been softening in the bath water, says Thibiant, a cool rinse is enough to wash them off and give you a very gentle, natural exfoliation. (Note: You should never soak longer than 20 minutes during any treatment or your birthday suit will start to dehydrate and turn raisinlike.)

- **Multitask with a mask.** Before you get into a warm bath, apply a thick layer of a clay face mask, and place a washcloth in a bowl of cool water near your tub. The bath's hot steam will help the mask absorb, and after 10 minutes, use the cool cloth to wipe away the clay and refresh your skin.

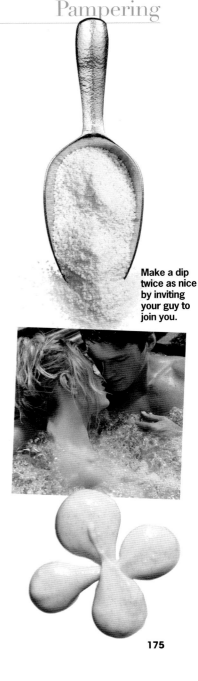

Make a dip twice as nice by inviting your guy to join you.

175

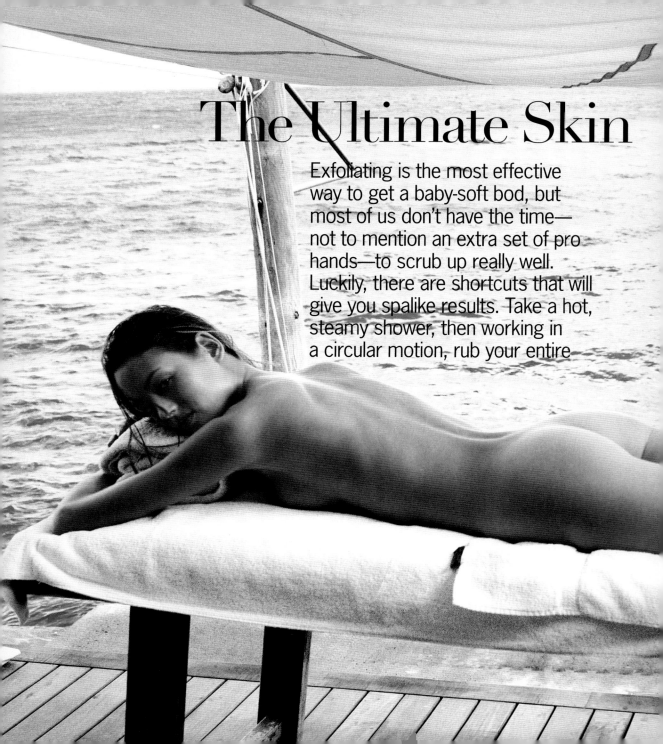

The Ultimate Skin

Exfoliating is the most effective way to get a baby-soft bod, but most of us don't have the time—not to mention an extra set of pro hands—to scrub up really well. Luckily, there are shortcuts that will give you spalike results. Take a hot, steamy shower, then working in a circular motion, rub your entire

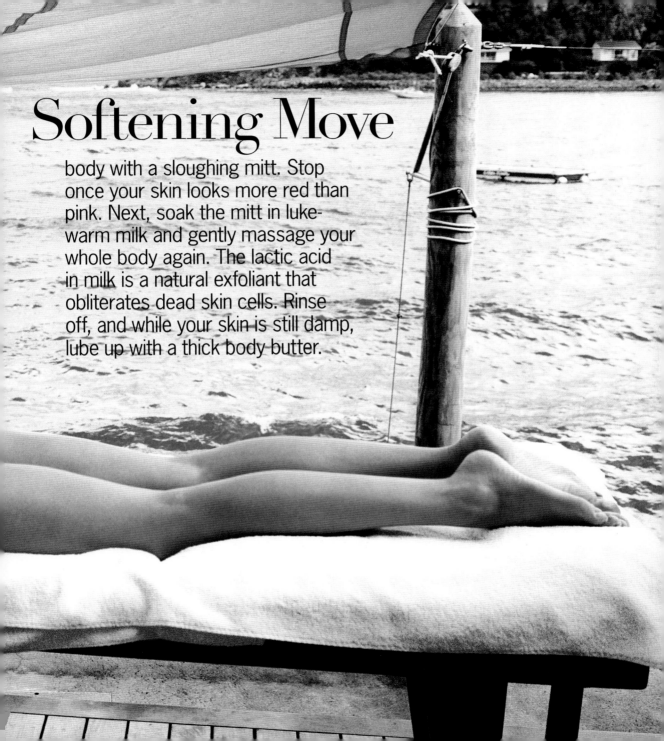

Softening Move

body with a sloughing mitt. Stop once your skin looks more red than pink. Next, soak the mitt in luke-warm milk and gently massage your whole body again. The lactic acid in milk is a natural exfoliant that obliterates dead skin cells. Rinse off, and while your skin is still damp, lube up with a thick body butter.

The Sexiest Spa Treatments on Earth

It's no secret that Cosmo likes anything exotic or erotic. And we've found a way to score both with some sensual head-to-toe pampering from all corners of the globe. "Many treatments from abroad rely on techniques that have been used for centuries to improve the body, skin, and hair," says Sue Harmsworth, CEO and founder of spa consultant and management company ESPA International. But amazingly, just about everything you need to replicate them is in your fridge or, even better, a pretty jar within close reach.

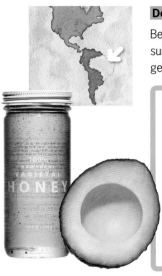

Destination Brazil

Being that some of the sexiest supermodels hail from this country, we're pretty sure Brazilians have a handle on all things beautiful. Their secret (besides great genes)? Slathering on fresh fruits and plants that help cleanse and moisturize.

Amazing Amazon Body Smoothie

Like those tasty beverages at the juice bar, this revitalizing skin "drink" is packed with antioxidants and vitamins that make you gleam.

- 2 c. full-fat plain yogurt ● ½ ripe avocado ● 5 large strawberries
- 2 T. honey ● 1 ripe banana

Whip all the ingredients in a blender. Apply the mix to your entire body and let it sit for 15 minutes. The vitamin C in this recipe helps brighten the skin, explains Shalini Vadhera, author of *Passport to Beauty*.

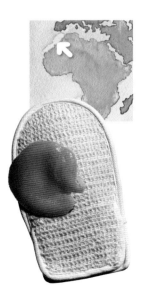

Destination Morocco

Morocco is a melting pot of African, French, Islamic, and Spanish cultures, so their spas incorporate a medley of exotic ingredients.

Seductive Steam Bath

Moroccan women swear by *hammams* to revitalize their bodies. Make this one a bit more romantic by asking your guy to help.
- Step into a supersteamy shower. Once your skin softens up a bit, move away from the water and apply a citrus-infused body scrub.
- Rinse and lather up with a rose-scented soap. The buds grow wild in the region, and the extracts help repair delicate skin, says Bill Toth, spa director at the Ballantyne Resort, in Charlotte, North Carolina. Finish by rubbing on a minty oil (another local favorite) to stay smooth.

India

This country has been inventing sexy moves since ancient times (kama sutra, anyone?). Their Ayurvedic spa rituals are just as tantalizing.

Tension-Ridding Rub

A traditional Ayurvedic massage begins with reading your dosha (body and mind type) to determine which essential oils match your needs, explains Holly Hatfield, spa director of the Chopra Center and Spa in NYC. Try rosemary for a pick-me-up, lavender if you're stressed, and rose before bedtime. Warm up a few drops of the oil in your hands before getting started.

Begin massaging the shoulders and work down to the toes, using broad strokes and applying medium pressure to relax the muscles.

Rub the joints (the sides of the hips, backs of the knees, and inner elbows) with open palms and circular motions—this is an Ayurvedic trick for increasing circulation, says Hatfield.

Make your feet tingle. Firmly run the open part of your hand back and forth over the soles.

A relaxed body is a beautiful one.

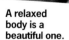

Stimulating Scalp Move

Women in India do weekly scalp massages to keep their hair shiny, says Vadhera. And since guys tend to carry stress in the neck area, this rejuvenating fix is good for them too.

Rub four or five drops of coconut or almond essential oil between your palms to warm it up.

Starting at the tip of the forehead, move your fingers back slowly (in small circular motions) toward the base of the neck.

Repeat for about 10 minutes, then have your guy return the favor.

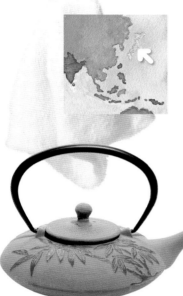

Destination Japan

The spas in this region have a Zen philosophy that cherishes serenity, says Tracy Okabe, from the Japanese-inspired spa Pola Kirei, in Santa Monica, California.

Refreshing Rice Soak

Japanese spas incorporate skin smoothers like rice and ginger into their baths. To create a sanctuary in your own tub:

Fire up a sandalwood candle; the scent is said to purify the air.

Fill your tub with lukewarm water, and add a few tablespoons of a rice soak. While you're in there, rub your entire body with a salt scrub to slough off dead cells. Start at your feet and work your way up.

Once you've rinsed off, apply a ginger-spiked body lotion while your skin is still damp. Let it absorb while you sip on a cup of green tea, Japan's Zen beverage of choice.

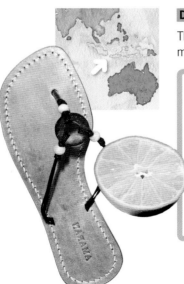

Destination Indonesia

This island nation is so rich in natural beauty ingredients that spas often mash stuff in front of you, then apply it straight to your body.

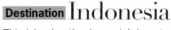

The Far East Foot Scrub

It's always sandal season in Indonesia, so women there know how to keep their toes in shape. To follow in their footsteps:

Cut a lime in half and rub your feet with it.

Slather on a mud mask to soothe.

Wash it off, pat your feet dry, and paint your toenails with a hue inspired by Indonesian batik (a vibrant textile), like sunset orange or red.

What Guys Love (and Hate) About Your Beauty Habits

It's easy to assume that men are totally oblivious to how much effort women put into their beauty routines.

But most dudes are way more observant than you think. And not only do they pay attention to your primping proclivities, they have opinions about them. Need proof? Read on for quotes from real guys.

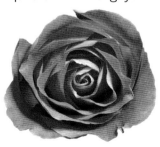

■ Fragrance

"My girlfriend mostly wears perfume for our weekend dates. So when I catch just the slightest whiff of it at any other time, it immediately conjures up an image of her in high heels and tight jeans." —*Kurt. 26*

"When I first laid eyes on my girlfriend, I wasn't sure I'd be into her because she's reserved. But when I got a little closer I smelled this exotic, musky perfume and that convinced me that she must have a daring side lurking beneath the conservative exterior." —*Henry, 26*

"I once had an innocent crush on a girl who wore this amazing floral scent. After I hugged her good-bye one day, the scent rubbed off on my scarf and lingered for days. Every time I smelled it, I kept thinking about being with her and kissing her. It drove me crazy, to the point where I actually broke up with the girl I was dating at the time to pursue the one who smelled so good." —*Marco, 31*

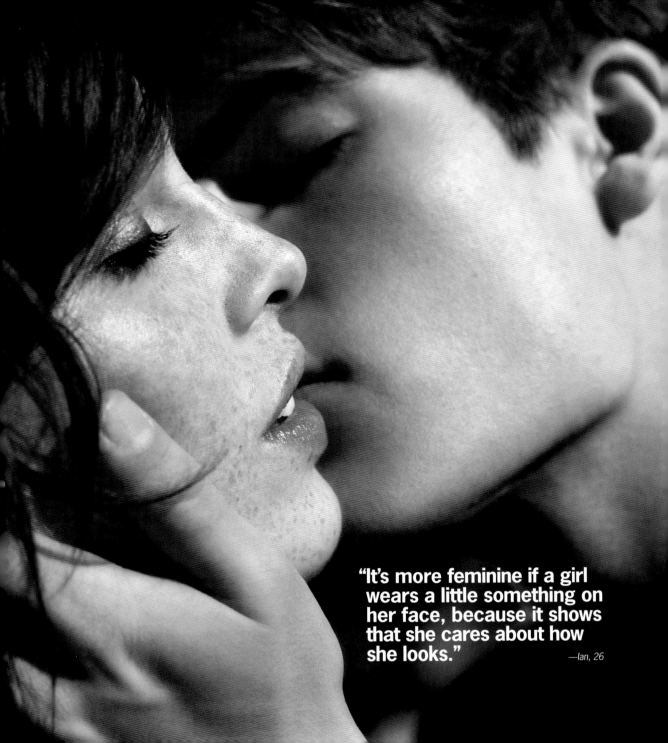

"It's more feminine if a girl wears a little something on her face, because it shows that she cares about how she looks."

—Ian, 26

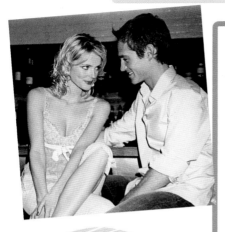

Sexy Surprise!
Try an unexpected move, like spraying perfume in your hair. Novelty drives up the brain's dopamine levels, which regulate arousal.

SOURCE: ANTHROPOLOGIST
HELEN FISHER, PHD

Guys can't keep their hands off a velvety bod.

■ Hair

"I am a sucker for women who can flirt with their hair. I still remember a girl I saw on the train six years ago. She glanced at me with one eye partially concealed by her hair. So mysterious." —Jeremy, 28

"It's so hot when a girl wears her hair up when we're out and then takes it down as soon as we're alone. It means she's totally comfortable with me and probably won't hold back in the sack." —Rob, 27

"There's nothing better than the phenomenal smell of freshly shampooed hair." —Benry, 22

"My girlfriend has naturally curly hair. She likes to straighten it, which looks good, but it's always such a turn-on when she leaves it all wild." —Jon, 22

"I think rumpled, slept-in bedhead is an incredibly appealing look on pretty much any woman." —Thomas, 25

■ Body

"Something magical must happen when girls step into the shower because they always come out with the silkiest, most amazing smelling skin imaginable." —Josh, 29

"I love feeling the supersoft skin on a girl's back. It gives me extra incentive to give her a massage." —Brent, 24

"When I'm lying in bed with a women and her legs are really smooth, it makes her body seem that much hotter." —Jeff, 26

■ Makeup

"Some juicy-looking lip gloss and long black eyelashes are better than if she has no makeup on at all. It's more feminine if a girl wears a little makeup because it shows that she cares about how she looks." —*Ian, 26*

"Nothing gets me worked up like those smoky bad-girl eyes." —*Rick, 28*

"I find the act of applying lipstick so sexy. It gets me thinking about what she can do with those lips." —*Tristan, 24*

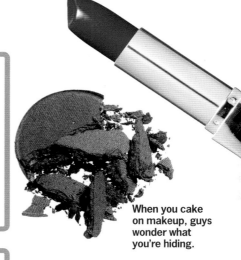

When you cake on makeup, guys wonder what you're hiding.

■ Nails

"I dig when girls keep their nails short and paint them a dark color, like red. It catches my attention." —*Brian, 29*

"The way I see it, if you care enough to be meticulous about your feet by painting your toenails, then I know you're taking good care of yourself in more private places." —*Jay, 22*

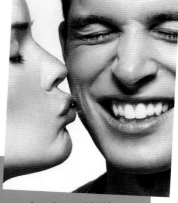

Not-So-Hot Beauty Moves

Some get-gorgeous practices drive guys crazy…in a bad way.

"I met a girl online who seemed really cool, so we decided to go out. But when she climbed into my car, I almost had an allergy attack. It smelled like she had just taken a bath in patchouli oil. I couldn't wait to drop her off so I could breathe again." —**David, 30**

"A blind date had the longest freakin' fingernails I've ever seen. She could barely pick up her knife and fork with those claws. Watching her stab at her cell phone keyboard put the absolute fear of God in me. There was no way I was going to let her near my most prized parts." —**Paul, 27**

"I went on a few dates with this chick who was obsessed with her hair. I ran my fingers through it when we were fooling around and my hand came out sticky. I don't know what the product was, but it smelled like paint remover." —**Kevin, 26**

A

Accutane, **26**
Acne, **24–27**
  on back and butt, **136**
  birth-control pills and, **26**
  blue-light therapy for, **26**
  chemical peels for, **26**
  cleansers and, **25**
  foundation fighting, **34**
  freezing out zits, **25**
  hiding, **25, 33**
  laser treatment for, **26**
  mild to moderate, treatments, **25**
  moisturizers and, **25**
  oily skin and, **12, 15**
  preventing and treating, **25–27, 136**
  regimen treatment time, **27**
  scars, **15, 20**
  severe, treatments, **26**
  spot treatments, **25**
  unclogging pores and, **13, 15, 25, 26, 136**
  using zit cream, **14**
  when to see dermatologist, **27**
African-American women
  biggest aging issues, **20**
  blush hues for, **37**
  bronzer on, **40**
  foundation considerations, **32**
  hair care tips, **88, 89**
  red nails for, **163**
Aging
  biggest issues by ethnicity, **20–21**
  fighting, **18–19**
Alpha-hydroxy acid, **13, 15, 18, 21, 169**
Amazon body smoothie (Brazil), **179**
Antioxidants, **18, 22, 179**
Antiperspirant, **137**
Arnold, Jan, **169**
Asian women
  biggest aging issues, **20**
  eye shadow tip, **55**
  foundation considerations, **32**

B

Baek, Ji, **160**
Barshop, Cindy, **128, 130, 131**
Bartolucci, Cristina, **36, 48**

Baths
  blissful, **174, 175**
  seductive steam, **179**
Beauty, sexy, **7**
Bikini line, **126–127**
Birth-control pills, **26**
Blandi, Oscar, **91**
Blow-drying hair, **89, 92–93**
Blue-light therapy, **26**
Blush
  applying, **36**
  colors by skin tone, **37**
  lasting, base for, **36**
  lighting-specific, **38–39**
  round-the-clock tips, **42–43**
Body, **120–139.** See also Legs
  beautifying your bust, **124–125**
  bikini line, **126–127**
  bling and sheen, **138–139**
  fixing bummers on, **136–137.** See also
    Acne
  his preferences, **184**
  moisturizing. See Moisturizers
  shimmer powder/cream, **134, 138, 139**
  sloughing, **123.** See also Exfoliating;
    Scrubbing skin; Scrubs
  sweat and antiperspirants, **137**
Brandt, Fredric, **12, 26**
Bronzer, **38, 40, 42, 43, 99, 124, 131**
Brown, Bobbi, **33**
Bruises, hiding, **137**
Buckingham, Peter, **83**
Bust
  beautifying, **124–125**
  breathable-fabric bras and, **137**
  preventing sweat around, **137**

C

Ceramides, **13**
Chemical peels, **15, 18, 20, 26**
Chocolate, **22**
Cilmi, Ann Marie, **128**
Cleansers
  daily regime, by skin type, **13**
  preventing acne, **25**
  usage (quantity) guidelines, **14**
Cleavage, accentuating, **124–125**

Cologne, effects of, **150.**
  See also Fragrance
Combination skin, **12, 13**
Complexion. See Skin
Concealer
  applying, **34**
  hiding dark circles, **64, 65**
Cunningham, Michael, **74**
Curling irons, **89**
Curry, Shannon, **175**
Cykiert, Robert, **61, 64**

D

Dakar, Sonya, **25, 73**
Daron, Nona, **138**
Day cream, **14**
DeVincenzo, Mark, **90**
Diet
  fragrance selection and, **145**
  omega-3 fatty acids and, **22**
  skin health and, **18, 22**
Dimples, outsmarting, **136**
Dorf, Paula, **58**
Dover, Jeffrey, **122**
Dry skin, **12, 13, 15**

E

Effleurage, **124**
Emich-Patton, Ann, **160**
Ethnic skin issues, **20–21.** See also African-
  American women; Asian women
Exfoliating, **15, 18, 130, 166, 175, 176–177.** See also Scrubbing skin; Scrubs
Eyebrows
  brushing, **62**
  choosing grooming method, **63**
  finding professional help, **63**
  as guide to hair color, **98**
  shaping, **62**
  thickening, **63**
  tinting, **63**
  trimming, **62**
  tweezing/waxing, **62, 63**
Eye cream, **14, 18, 20, 64**
Eyelashes
  curling, **60**
  fake, **61**

fatter, longer, denser, **60**
lower, coating, **60**
ultrasexy, **60–61**
Eyeliner
best looks, **58–59**
counteracting bloodshot eyes, **59, 64**
daytime and nighttime looks, **58**
enhancing lashes, **60**
making it last, **51**
pencil, powder, or liquid, **58**
smudgy look, **53**
sparkle, **58**
Eyes, **44–65**
bags under, deflating, **64**
best colors for, **48**
close-set, tips for, **55**
effects lasting longer, **50–51**
enlarging trick, **51**
hiding dark circles, **64, 65**
his thoughts on, **185**
hooded, tips for, **55**
preparing for makeup, **50**
problems solved, **64–65**
ridding redness, **59, 64**
small, tips for, **55**
sultry, evening, **52, 56–57**
tips for every shape, **55**
Eye shadow
applying, **50–51, 54–55**
brush selection, **54**
color of, eye color and, **48**
making it last longer, **50–51**
multiple effects with one hue, **54**
quad colors explained, **50**
shopping for, **49**
smoldering stare with, **56–57**
sultry, evening eyes, **52, 56–57**
tips for every eye shape, **55**
vibrant hues, **52**

F

Face. See Blush; Foundation; Makeup;
Moisturizers; Skin
Factor, Davis, **39**
Feet
at-home soak, **166**
daily care regime, **169**
DIY pedicure, **166–167, 168**
his thoughts on, **185**

Indonesian foot scrub, **181**
nail color by time of year, **168**
waxing hair on piggies, **167**
Fisher, Helen, **79, 184**
Flavored lotions, **138**
Foot scrubs, **166, 169, 181**
Foundation
applying, **33, 34**
as concealer, **35**
finding right shade, **32**
getting more from, **35**
shopping for, **32**
types of, for varying conditions, **34**
Fragrance, **140–155**
affecting your attitude, **154**
citrus and fruits, **144, 146**
creating, **154**
effects of different aromas, **144**
excessive, avoiding, **152, 155, 185**
florals, **144, 146**
forespraying lingerie, **152**
forms of, **described, 147**
gourmands, **144**
his, affecting you, **150**
his preferences, **145, 182, 185**
importance of, **142**
making it last, **153**
mood-defining quiz, **146**
mysterious, adventurous, or wildly
romantic, **146**
orientals and musks, **144, 146**
pulse points for, **152, 153**
right, finding, **145**
scent/seduction link, **148**
shopping for, **145**
solid, **147**
tricks to flaunt, **152–153**
where to wear, **152**
Freezing out zits, **25**
French manicure, **164**
Fusco, Francesca, **42, 43**

G

Gafni, Ramy, **55, 62**
Gambill, Kimberly, **174**
Geller, Laura, **58**
Gibson, Ted, **90**
Gilbert, Avery, **150**

Giordano, Susan, **70**
Givens, David, **46, 125**
Graf, Jeannette, **126, 128, 130, 131, 166**
Guys, **182–185**
attraction to lips, **79, 81, 83, 185**
cologne, affecting you, **150**
fragrance preferences, **145, 182, 185**
on hair, **184, 185**
on makeup, **183, 185**
on nails, **185**
not-so-hot moves for, **185**
red lips affecting, **81**
scent/seduction link, **148**
shaving down there and, **127**
on skin and smoothness, **184**

H

Hadley, Skyy, **164**
Hair, **84–117.** See also Bikini line; Legs
adding volume to, **90–91**
African-American, **tips, 88, 89**
blow-drying, **89, 92–93**
brushes, **88**
curling irons, **89**
deep side part, **94**
detangling, **88**
disasters. See Hair disaster repair
gloss treatments, **90, 101**
headband or scarf in, **94**
healthy, strategies, **88–90**
heating precautions, **89**
his thoughts on, **184, 185**
lazy updo, **95**
massaging head and, **88**
posh ponytail, **94**
quick-styling tips, **94–95**
reviving day-out blowout, **95**
reviving roots, **95**
shiny, hints for, **90, 92**
split ends Rx, **88**
styles. See Hairstyles
and quick switches
Velcro rollers for, **91, 95**
washing, **88, 90, 101**
Hair color
blond for dark skin, **98**
blond highlights enhancing complexion, **98**
brow color guiding, **98**
darkening, **100**

finding perfect hue, **98–99**
fixing dud dye job, **96**
highlights, **98, 101**
lightening, **100**
pro job at home, **100–101**
protecting and preserving, **101**
touching up roots, **100**
Hair disaster repair, **96–97**
bad bang trim, **97**
dud dye job, **96**
hat hair, **96**
product overload, **97**
Hairstyles and quick switches, **102–117**
about: highlighting your best features,
110; picking stylist, **105;** working with
stylists, **110, 117**
Beautiful Backsweep, **107**
Bedhead Waves, **105**
Boho Waves, **110**
Chic Bob, **112**
Foxy Fringe, **111**
Full-On Curls, **106**
Messy Bun, **114**
Modern Pixie, **108**
Pretty Plait, **109**
Relaxed Pony, **113**
Sexy Blowback, **115**
Shaggy Crop, **116**
Sleek Blunt Cut, **104**
Sultry Braid, **117**
Sweet Spirals, **102–103**
Hands. See also Nails
massaging, **160**
nighttime pampering treatment, **160**
Harler, Jason, **174**
Harmsworth, Sue, **178**
Hatfield, Holly, **180**
Hatton, Susie, **131**
Haviland-Jones, Jeannette, **148**
Hay, Linda, **134**
Hazen, Rita, **98, 100**
Heftler, Noah S., **16**
Herbert, Lisa, **81**
Herz, Rachel, **152**
Hickeys, hiding, **136**
Hirsch, Alan, **144, 147, 148, 152**
Hispanic aging issues, **21**
Hyperpigmentation, **20**

I
Ingrown hairs, **126**

K
Kelly, Maureen, **49**
Kidd, Jemma, **33, 36, 40**
Kudia, Scott, **74**
Kunin, Audrey, **137**

L
Laser treatment, **26**
Legs
beauty tricks, **134**
bikini line, **126–127**
bumps and "chicken skin," **126, 137**
his preferences, **184**
self-tanning, **130–133, 134**
shaping bikini line, **127**
shaving, **126, 128–129**
slimming and lengthening
look of, **134–135**
smoother longer, **128**
waxing, **127, 128, 167**
Lemon, for skin, **124, 174**
Lighting, makeup and, **38–39**
Lip gloss, **70, 72, 73, 77, 78, 185**
Lip liner, **72, 78**
Lippmann, Deborah, **161, 164**
Lips, **66–83**
applying color, **76**
come-hither shades for, **82**
dark lipstick hint, **80**
fuller mouth without
makeup, **72**
his attraction to, **79, 83, 185**
homemade mask for, **71**
invisible liner for, **78**
keeping color off teeth, **76**
lasting color for, **78**
lusty, **82**
plumping, **72–73**
priming, for color, **70, 76, 78**
protecting from sun, **70**
scarlet tones, sexy
appeal of, **80–81**
seduction secret, **74**
smooch-proofing color, **78**
testing colors for, in store, **76**

Logan, Alan C., **22**
Longo, Vincent, **73**

M
Makeup. See also Blush; Eye shadow;
Eyeliner; Foundation; Mascara
bronzer, **38, 40, 42, 43, 99, 124, 131**
fuller mouth without, **72**
his preferences, **183, 185**
lighting-specific, **38–39**
for morning/evening,
weekday/weekend, **42–43**
orgasmic facial flush and, **38**
round-the-clock tips, **42–43**
shades, importance of, **30**
Manicure. See Nails
Mascara
applying, **60, 61**
eye-enlarging trick, **51**
on lower lashes, **60**
making it last, **51**
for small and close-set eyes, **55**
Masks, **71, 124, 175, 181**
Massage, **88, 174, 175, 177, 180**
Matin, **40, 64**
McDonald, Marguerite, **64**
Moisturizers
acne and, **25**
applying, **12, 18, 122**
daily use, by skin type, **13**
day cream, **14**
flavored, **138**
locking in moisture, **122**
night cream, **14, 21**
optimizing, **12, 14, 122**
tinted, liquid highlighter in, **41**
types of, **13**
usage (quantity) guidelines, **14, 18, 122**
Molnar, Theresa, **154**
Monahan, Gretchen, **123**
Mordini, Holly, **38, 51**
Murad, Howard, **136**

N
Nails, **156–169.** See also Feet
broken, fixing, **160**
flawless paint job, **163**
French manicure, **164**

his preferences, **185**
importance of, **158**
polish pointers, **164–165**
pro manicure techniques, **161**
reds for, **162–163**
shapes and shaping, **161**
Nigara, Mathew, **80**
Night cream, **14, 21**
Normal skin, **12, 13**

O

Oily skin, **12, 13, 15**
Okabe, Tracy, **181**
Ophals, Gabrielle, **127**
Osmond, Polly, **51**

P

Pampering yourself. *See* Spa secrets
Patterson, Blair, **58**
Pedicure. *See* Feet
Perillo, Donna, **166**
Pimples. See Acne
Pores
    large, diminishing, **15**
    skin type and, **12**
    unclogging, **13, 15, 25, 26, 136**
Pozzetti, Nicole, **124**

Q

Queen, Carol, **127**

R

Retinoid, **18, 26**
Retinol, **18, 21, 25**
Rice soak (Japan), **181**
Roncal, Mally, **54, 60, 64, 72, 82**

S

Salicylic acid, **13, 25, 34, 126, 136**
Sanders, Chantal, **136**
Scalp massage, **88, 174, 180**
Scents. See Fragrance
Sciales, Christopher, **12, 15, 18, 22**
Scrubbing skin, **123, 130, 137,
160, 166**
Scrubs, **15, 122, 124, 137,
169, 179, 181**

Self-tanning, **130–133, 134**
Serquinia, Julie, **166**
Sexy beauty, defined, **7**
Shaving, **126, 128–129**
Shaw, Carol, **32, 36, 72**
Showers, soothing, **174**
Siegel, Robin, **52**
Silicone, **13, 90, 128**
Skin, **8–27**. *See also* Acne
    aging issues by ethnicity, **20–22**
    cleansing, **13**
    combination, **12, 13**
    daily care regime, **13**
    diet, nutrition and, **18, 22**
    dry, **12, 13, 15**
    exfoliating, **15, 18, 130, 157,
        166, 176–177**. *See also* Scrubbing
        skin; Scrubs
    fighting aging, **18–19**
    his preferences, **184**
    key to glowing complexion, **10**
    lemon for, **124, 174**
    normal, **12, 13**
    oily, **12, 13, 15**
    pampering. See Spa secrets
    sleep and, **22, 43**
    sun protection, **16**
    supermarket smoothers for, **124**
    tones, perfect reds for, **163**
    types and characteristics, **12**
    vitamins and, **18, 20, 22, 179**
Skin products. See also Moisturizers
    cleansers, **13, 14**
    daily care, **13**
    usage (quantity) guidelines, **14**
Sleep, **22, 43**
Sloughing. *See* Exfoliating; Scrubbing skin
Spa secrets, **170–181**
    Amazon body smoothie (Brazil), **179**
    from around the world, **178–181**
    blissful baths, **174, 175**
    exfoliating, **15, 176–177**. *See also*
        Scrubs
    foot scrub (Indonesia), **181**
    rice soak (Japan), **181**
    scalp massage (India), **180**
    seductive steam bath (Morocco), **179**

sensual aromas, **174**
    soothing showers, **174**
    tension-ridding rub (India), **180**
    watsu massage, **175**
    Steam bath (Morocco), **179**
Strong, Collier, **38**
Sun protection, **16–17, 19, 20, 21, 70**
Sunspots, **20**
Surratt, Troy, **33**
Sweat, antiperspirant and, **137**

T

Tahmasebi, Cyrus, **77**
Tanned look
    bronzer and, **40**
    self-tanning, **130–133, 134**
Tanzi, Elizabeth, **122**
Teeth, looking brighter, **77**
Thibiant, Aida, **175**
Tiger, Lionel, **38, 162**
Tilbury, Charlotte, **40**
Toth, Bill, **179**
Turnbow, Tina, **34**
Twine, Judy, **60**

V

Vadhera, Shalini, **179, 180**
Vartoughian, Jessica, **161**
Vitamins, **18, 20, 22, 179**
Vitello, Denise, **122**

W

Warren, Craig, **144**
Watsu massage, **175**
Waxing, **127, 128, 167**
Weingarten, Essie, **168**
White, Soren, **10**
Wild, Debbie, **154**
Williams, Patricia Yankee, **160**
Wilson, Ni'Kita, **128**
Wrinkles, **16, 21, 22**

Z

Zicu, Cornelia, **71, 123**
Zits. *See* Acne
Zomnir, Wende, **50**

■ Cover and Title Page

Cliff Watts (Cover stills) Svend Lindbaek; Jeffrey Westbrook/Studio D.; Chris Eckert/Studio D. (Back cover models) Peter Buckingham; Michael Williams; David Stesner; Chris Fortuna

■ Table of Contents

PAGE 4: Butch Hogan

PAGE 5: Svend Lindbaek (4); Peter Buckingham

■ Intro

PAGES 12 to 13: Jeff Lipsky

■ Skin

PAGE 9: Peter Buckingham

PAGE 11: David Stesner

PAGE 12: Jack Miskell; Svend Lindbaek; Jack Miskell; Svend Lindbaek

PAGE 13: David Stesner

PAGE 14: Roger Cabello; Svend Lindbaek (4)

PAGE 15: Svend Lindbaek; Greg Broom

PAGE 16: Jack Miskell; Myers Robertson

PAGE 17: Marc Baptiste

PAGE 18: Svend Lindbaek

PAGE 19: Todd Marshard

PAGE 20: Viki Forshee; Greg Sorensen

PAGE 21: Peter Buckingham; Myers Robertson

PAGE 22: Svend Lindbaek; Jeffrey Westbrook/Studio D.; Jack Miskell

PAGE 23: Jeff Olson

PAGE 24: Chris Eckert/Studio D.

PAGE 25: Roger Cabello; Svend Lindbaek (2); Marc Baptiste

PAGE 26: David Turner/Studio D.; Jeff Lipsky

PAGE 27: Dennis Golonka

■ Face

PAGE 29: David Stesner

PAGE 31: Jeff Olson

PAGE 32: Svend Lindbaek

PAGE 33: Svend Lindbaek; Todd Barry

PAGE 34: Svend Lindbaek; Jeffrey Westbrook/Studio D.; Svend Lindbaek (2); Peter Buckingham

PAGE 35: Svend Lindbaek

PAGE 36: Svend Lindbaek

PAGE 37: Greg Sorensen (2); Marc Baptiste; Chris Eckert/Studio D. (3); Svend Lindbaek (2); Chris Eckert/Studio D.

PAGE 38: Svend Lindbaek; Jeffrey Westbrook/Studio D.

PAGE 39: Todd Marshard

PAGE 40: Chris Eckert/Studio D.; Svend Lindbaek; (compact) Jeffrey Westbrook/Studio D.; (makeup) Roger Cabello

PAGE 41: Chris Fortuna

PAGE 42: Peter Buckingham; Chris Eckert/Studio D. (2)

PAGE 43: Svend Lindbaek; Roxanne Lowit; Svend Lindbaek

■ Eyes

PAGE 45: Peter Buckingham

PAGE 47: Marc Baptiste

PAGE 48: Svend Lindbaek; Jeffrey Westbrook/Studio D. (2); Svend Lindbaek (3)

PAGE 49: Jeffrey Westbrook/Studio D.

PAGE 50: Jeffrey Westbrook/Studio D.; Ben Perini; Roger Cabello

PAGE 51: Jeffrey Westbrook/Studio D.; Svend Lindbaek (2).

PAGE 52: Eric Fischer; Ben Perini (2)

PAGE 53: Kelly Ryerson

PAGE 54: Svend Lindbaek (3); Peter Buckingham

PAGE 55: Ben Perini

PAGE 57: Dean Isidro

PAGE 58: Roger Cabello; Marc Baptiste; Nicola Majocchi; Svend Lindbaek

PAGE 59: Eliston Lutz

PAGE 60-: Svend Lindbaek; Chris Eckert/Studio D.; Eric Fischer

PAGE 61: Jeffrey Westbrook/Studio D.

PAGE 62: Jeffrey Westbrook/Studio D.; Ben Perini; Marko Metzinger/Studio D.

PAGE 63: Peter Buckingham; Roger Cabello

PAGE 64: Roger Cabello; Ben Perini; Svend Lindbaek

PAGE 65: Anna Palma

■ Lips

PAGE 67: Marc Baptiste

PAGE 69: Dean Isidro

PAGE 70: Jeffrey Westbrook/Studio D.; Jack Miskell; Jeffrey Westbrook/Studio D.; Tamara Schlesinger

PAGE 71: Jeffrey Westbrook/Studio D.

PAGE 72: Svend Lindbaek (2); Ben Perini

PAGE 73: Jeffrey Westbrook/Studio D.

PAGE 75: Chris Fortuna

PAGE 76: Svend Lindbaek

PAGE 77: Marc Baptiste

PAGE 78: Svend Lindbaek; Walter Sassard

PAGE 79: Chris Fortuna

PAGE 80: Jeffrey Westbrook/Studio D.

PAGE 81: Chris Eckert/Studio D.; Nicola Majocchi

PAGE 82: Svend Lindbaek (4); Eric Fischer

PAGE 83: Kelly Ryerson

■ Hair

PAGE 85: Eric Fischer

PAGE 87: David Stesner

PAGE 88: Svend Lindbaek

PAGE 89: David Stesner; Svend Lindbaek; Todd Barry

PAGE 90: Svend Lindbaek

PAGE 91: Cliff Watts (4)

PAGE 92: Roger Cabello; Svend Lindbaek (2)

PAGE 93: Dean Isidro

PAGE 94: Dean Isidro; Jeffrey Westbrook/ Studio D.; Marc Baptiste

PAGE 95: Svend Lindbaek; Chris Fortuna; Svend Lindbaek

PAGE 96: Marc Baptiste

PAGE 97: Peter Buckingham; Roger Cabello; Svend Lindbaek

PAGE 98: Svend Lindbaek

PAGE 99: Marc Baptiste

PAGE 101: Butch Hogan; Svend Lindbaek (2)

PAGE 102-103: Alex Freund

PAGE 104: Marc Baptiste

PAGE 105: Ben Shaul

PAGE 106: Michael Williams

PAGE 107: Eric Fischer

PAGE 108: Eric Fischer

PAGE 109: Dean Isidro

PAGE 110: Marc Baptiste

PAGE 111: Peter Buckingham

PAGE 112: Thom Eichinger

PAGE 113: Butch Hogan

PAGE 114: Butch Hogan

PAGE 115: Marc Baptiste

PAGE 116: Thom Eichinger

PAGE 117: Eric Fischer

Body

PAGE 119: Chris Fortuna

PAGE 121: Patrick Demarchelier

PAGE 122: fotosearch.com; Marc Baptiste

PAGE 123: Svend Lindbaek

PAGE 124: Svend Lindbaek

PAGE 125: Marc Baptiste

PAGE 126: Svend Lindbaek

PAGE 127: Jeffrey Westbrook/Studio D.; Svend Lindbaek

PAGE 128: Svend Lindbaek

PAGE 129: Chris Fortuna

PAGE 130: Svend Lindbaek

PAGE 131: Roger Cabello; Alex Freund

PAGES 132 to 133: Todd Marshard

PAGE 134: Chris Eckert/Studio D. (Illustrations) Chico Hayashi/cwc-i.com

PAGE 135: Chris Fortuna

PAGE 136: Svend Lindbaek; Tamara Schlesinger

PAGE 137: Kevin Sweeney/Studio D.; Svend Lindbaek

PAGE 138: Svend Lindbaek

PAGE 139: Greg Sorensen

Fragrance

PAGE 141: Jeff Olson

PAGE 143: Chris Fortuna

PAGE 144: Svend Lindbaek

PAGE 145: Kelly Ryerson

PAGE 146: Svend Lindbaek

PAGE 147: Svend Lindbaek

PAGE 149: Chris Fortuna

PAGE 151: Kelly Ryerson

PAGE 152: Chris Fortuna

PAGE 153: Svend Lindbaek

PAGE 154: Svend Lindbaek; Jeffrey Westbrook/Studio D.

PAGE 155: Marc Baptiste

Nails

PAGE 157: Peter Buckingham

PAGE 159: Jeff Olson

PAGE 160: Chris Eckert/Studio D.

PAGE 161: Svend Lindbaek; Ben Perini (3)

PAGE 162: Svend Lindbaek

PAGE 163: Chris Eckert/Studio D. (2); Roger Cabello; Ben Perini (2)

PAGE 164: Svend Lindbaek

PAGE 165: David Stesner

PAGE 166: Svend Lindbaek; Chris Eckert/ Studio D.; Roger Cabello (2)

PAGE 167: Greg Broom

PAGE 168: (Shimmery nail colors) Svend Lindbaek; (matte nail colors) Jeffrey Westbrook/Studio D.

PAGE 169: Roger Cabello; Svend Lindbaek; Roger Cabello

Pampering

PAGE 171: Kelly Ryerson

PAGE 173: Myers Robertson

PAGE 174: Svend Lindbaek; Roger Cabello

PAGE 175: Svend Lindbaek; Peter Buckingham; Svend Lindbaek

PAGES 176 to 177: Patrick Demarchelier

PAGE 178: Svend Lindbaek

PAGE 179: Svend Lindbaek (2); Roger Cabello

PAGE 180: Todd Marshard; Chris Eckert/ Studio D.

PAGE 181: Chris Eckert/Studio D.

Guy Section

PAGE 182: Svend Lindbaek

PAGE 183: Eric Cahan

PAGE 184: Roxanne Lowit; Roger Cabello

PAGE 185: Chris Eckert/Studio D.; Svend Lindbaek; Peter Buckingham

The models photographed in *Cosmo's Sexiest Beauty Secrets* are used for illustrative purposes only; *Cosmo's Sexiest Beauty Secrets* does not suggest that the models actually engage in the conduct discussed in the stories they illustrate.

COSMOPOLITAN

PROJECT DIRECTOR John Searles
TEXT BY Andrea Lavinthal
EDITED BY Michele Promaulayko
BOOK DESIGN BY Peter Perron
ASSOCIATE BEAUTY EDITOR Heather Muir
MANAGING EDITOR Seth Wharton

EDITOR-IN-CHIEF Kate White
DESIGN DIRECTOR Ann P. Kwong

Library of Congress Cataloging-in-Publication Data

Cosmo's Sexiest Beauty Secrets : The Ultimate Guide to Looking Gorgeous / from the Editors of Cosmopolitan. -- 1st paperback ed.
    p. cm.

Includes bibliographical references and index.
ISBN 978-1-58816-725-5 (alk. paper)
1. Beauty, Personal. 2. Feminine beauty (Aesthetics) 3. Beauty culture. 4. Cosmetics. I. Cosmopolitan (New York, N.Y. : 1952)
HQ1219.C67 2008
646.7'042--dc22   2008010642

10 9 8 7 6 5 4 3 2 1

Published by Hearst Books
A Division of Sterling Publishing Co., Inc.
387 Park Avenue South, New York, NY 10016

Cosmopolitan and Hearst Books are trademarks of Hearst Communications, Inc.

www.cosmopolitan.com

For information about custom editions, special sales, premium and corporate purchases, please contact Sterling Special Sales Department at 800-805-5489 or specialsales@sterlingpublishing.com.

Distributed in Canada by Sterling Publishing
c/o Canadian Manda Group, 165 Dufferin Street
Toronto, Ontario, Canada M6K 3H6

Distributed in Australia by Capricorn Link (Australia) Pty. Ltd.
P.O. Box 704, Windsor, NSW 2756 Australia

Manufactured in China

Sterling ISBN: 978-1-58816-725-5